Building Language Using
LEGO® Bricks

of related interest

LEGO®-Based Therapy
How to build social competence through LEGO®-Based Clubs for children with autism and related conditions
Daniel B. LeGoff, Gina Gómez de la Cuesta,
GW Krauss, and Simon Baron-Cohen
ISBN 978 1 84905 537 6
eISBN 978 0 85700 960 9

Talk to Me
Conversation Strategies for Parents of Children on the Autism Spectrum or with Speech and Language Impairments
Heather Jones
ISBN 978 1 84905 428 7
eISBN 978 0 85700 898 5

Music, Language and Autism
Exceptional Strategies for Exceptional Minds
Adam Ockelford
ISBN 978 1 84905 197 2
eISBN 978 0 85700 428 4

Speak, Move, Play and Learn with Children on the Autism Spectrum
Activities to Boost Communication Skills, Sensory Integration and Coordination Using Simple Ideas from Speech and Language Pathology and Occupational Therapy
Lois Jean Brady, America X Gonzalez, Maciej Zawadzki and Corinda Presley
ISBN 978 1 84905 872 8
eISBN 978 0 85700 531 1

Building Language Using LEGO® Bricks

A Practical Guide

Dawn Ralph and Jacqui Rochester

Foreword by Gina Gómez de la Cuesta

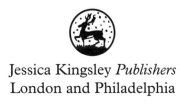

Jessica Kingsley *Publishers*
London and Philadelphia

First published in 2016
by Jessica Kingsley Publishers
73 Collier Street
London N1 9BE, UK
and
400 Market Street, Suite 400
Philadelphia, PA 19106, USA

www.jkp.com

Library of Congress Cataloging in Publication Data
Names: Ralph, Dawn.
Title: Building language using Lego bricks : a practical guide / Dawn Ralph and Jacqui Rochester ; foreword by Gina Gomez De La Cuesta.
Description: Philadelphia : Jessica Kingsley Publishers, 2016.
Identifiers: LCCN 2016007939 | ISBN 9781785920615 (alk. paper)
Subjects: LCSH: Autistic children--Education. | Autistic children--Language. | LEGO toys. | Communicative disorders in children.
Classification: LCC LC4717.85 .R35 2016 | DDC 371.94--dc23
LC record available at http://lccn.loc.gov/2016007939

British Library Cataloguing in Publication Data
A CIP catalogue record for this book is available from the British Library

ISBN 978 1 78592 061 5
eISBN 978 1 78450 317 8

Printed and bound in Great Britain

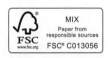

Contents

Conclusion 115

Foreword

I am delighted to write this foreword for *Building Language Using LEGO® Bricks*. I first encountered Jacqui Rochester, an autism specialist, and Dawn Ralph, a Speech and Language Therapist, when we exchanged emails about LEGO®-based therapy in 2010. These two talented professionals have since acquired a wealth of experience in using LEGO®-bricks to support young people with language impairment. In this book they share their expertise in adapting LEGO®-based therapy for this purpose. The book is creative, practical and thought-provoking and will be invaluable to Speech and Language Therapists, parents and other professionals wishing to support children with a wide range of language and communication problems.

I first became involved with LEGO®-based therapy during my PhD at the Autism Research Centre at the University of Cambridge. While working with Professor Simon Baron-Cohen and Dr Ayla Humphrey, I had the opportunity to visit Philadelphia, USA, to learn about LEGO®-based therapy from its pioneer, 'Dr Dan' LeGoff. Little did I know when I published my research back in 2008 that LEGO®-based therapy would prove to be such a popular and effective intervention. It is now widely used in schools and clinics across the UK, as well as internationally, to help young people with autism and other social communication difficulties to improve their social skills. I am thrilled to see LEGO®-based therapy being used to improve these young people's lives. The popularity of the approach, I believe, is down to the inherent appeal of LEGO® bricks and the fact that people are seeing positive results.

Building Language Using LEGO® Bricks takes LEGO®-based therapy in a new and important direction. In this practical guide, you can learn in detail about how to use LEGO® bricks to help children with even the most severe receptive and expressive language difficulties. The authors provide clear descriptions of different language and communication difficulties and outline exactly how adult facilitators can use LEGO® bricks to support children develop in a wide range of speech and language abilities. The approach can be individually tailored to the personal strengths and difficulties of the child. Targets for intervention range from developing joint attention and listening skills to understanding early concepts (such as size, colour, position and shape) or repairing communication breakdown. They provide comprehensive resources and a clear facilitator guide so that you have all you need to get started. Helpful and detailed case studies illustrate the important principles of using LEGO® bricks in this way, as well as highlighting the range of verbal and social communication difficulties that can be targeted.

When I train professionals in how to run LEGO®-based therapy, I am frequently asked how the approach can be adapted to young people who have additional learning difficulties or speech and language problems. From now on, I will be delighted to refer them to this comprehensive and thoughtful book. I hope that by publishing this methodology, research and evaluation of the impact of this approach will follow.

Overall, this book will help any reader understand how to harness the myriad uses of LEGO® bricks to develop communication with the young people they support. I congratulate the authors on their dedication, innovation and creativity!

Gina Gómez de la Cueste
Trainee Clinical Psychologist, University of
East Anglia and founder of Bricks for Autism,
LEGO-based therapy training courses

Acknowledgements

Our warmest thanks to the following people.

Our families for supporting us and understanding that while writing this we have seen more of each other than we have of them.

All the children and their families who have taught us so much over the years.

Jenny Meteyard for her patience and meticulous proofreading skills.

Allison Hope-West for her support and knowledge.

Gina Gómez de la Cuesta for her inspiration, support and encouragement.

Preface

I've just read an exciting article in the National Autistic Society's *Communication* magazine. I think we should give it a go! (Jacqui Rochester)

This was our introduction to using LEGO® bricks as a medium for therapy; the beginning of a massive learning curve for us and a powerful intervention tool for the wonderful young people we work with.

Having read the article (National Autistic Society, 2009) and decided to run our first ever group, we then struggled to find out exactly what to do. There was very little on the internet at the time. The only references we found were the original articles written by Dr LeGoff (2004), from the United States of America, and subsequent studies by the Autism Research Centre team (Owens *et al.*, 2008) in Cambridge. These were fascinating but added little to our knowledge of what we had to actually do.

Jacqui then contacted Gina Gómez de la Cuesta (née Owens) who very kindly sent through a PowerPoint presentation that gave us ideas on how to run sessions using LEGO® bricks in our therapy sessions.

This then became the basis for our initial attempts. These have been modified over time, as we have gained a better understanding of how this tool can be differentiated to meet the needs of a range of young people.

This book will describe how we have developed our practice from the original format into what we now call Building Language Using LEGO® Bricks.

It is intended to be a practical guide to enable both professionals and parents to set up and run Building Language Using LEGO®

Bricks sessions. We hope that sharing our experiences will empower readers to use this approach confidently and feel able to adapt it to meet a wider range of needs.

We will describe a Building Language Using LEGO® Bricks session and provide resources for your use and tools to baseline and help measure the efficacy of your intervention.

We will, of course, make reference to the research that inspired us in the first place, but the intention of this book is to be a practical and user-friendly guide for all to access. We will also include some of the reasons why we believe Building Language Using LEGO® Bricks works and how it taps into areas that other interventions have difficulty in reaching. Those readers who wish for a more in-depth knowledge of the theoretical basis and development of the original approach are directed to the reference for *LEGO®-Based Therapy* (LeGoff *et al.*, 2014) in the references section of this book.

This intervention has been used with a range of children and adults. As most of our clinical experience has been with children we have referred to participants in the intervention as 'the child' or 'children'. However, we have trained professionals who have used this approach with adults.

A brief description of Building Language Using LEGO® Bricks

Building Language Using LEGO® Bricks is a division-of-labour task, which takes the form of a barrier game. Two children work together to build a model. Each child has a specific role. One is the engineer, who has the instructions and relays these to the other child, the builder. The builder selects the correct bricks and places them on the model. The builder does not see the instructions but has to rely on directions from the engineer. Children experience both roles during a session. This division of labour means it is essential to work together to achieve a build.

An adult takes the role of a 'facilitator', helping the children to work together and use appropriate language and social communication skills. How they do this forms the majority of the content of this book.

Chapter 1

What Are Autism and Language Impairment?

What is autism?

The National Autistic Society (2016a) states that:

> Autism is a lifelong developmental disability that affects
> how a person communicates with, and relates to, other
> people. It also affects how they make sense of the world
> around them.

For many years, to receive a diagnosis of autism a person would
have displayed impairments in the following areas, known as the
'Triad of Impairments' (Wing and Gould, 1979):

- communication and language

- flexibility of thinking and behaviour

- social and emotional understanding.

These areas were classified under the Diagnostic and Statistical
Manual-IV (DSM-IV) (American Psychiatric, 1994) and the
International Classification of Diseases-10 (ICD-10) (World
Health Organization, 1993) and used as the criteria for a diagnosis
of autism.

In 2013, the Diagnostic and Statistical Manual was revised
by the American Psychiatric Association (APA) and the criteria
for diagnosis were changed (American Psychiatric Association,
2013). The new DSM-5, as it is known, reduced the three areas of
impairment to two.

The following is taken from the National Autistic Society's (2016b) description for the DSM-5, as it simplifies a complex definition into one that is easy to read and understand:

> The two areas are now:
>
> - social communication and interaction
> - restricted, repetitive patterns of behaviour, interests or activities (including sensory behaviours).

Under the DSM-5, the terms 'Asperger's Disorder', 'Childhood Disintegrative Disorder', 'Autistic Disorder' and 'Pervasive Developmental Disorder Not Otherwise Specified (PDD-NOS)' are no longer given as separate diagnoses. If the criteria are met, a single diagnosis of 'Autism Spectrum Disorder' (ASD) is used.

Autism is a 'spectrum' condition. The term 'spectrum' encompasses a wide range of skills and needs, from those who have no additional learning difficulties to those whose learning difficulties would be classed as severe. Some people with autism will go through their whole lives living independent lives without a diagnosis. Others will have lifelong dependency on carers.

For the entire range of the spectrum people with autism see and experience the world differently. It is not the wrong way or the right way, but it is a completely different way. These experiences can sometimes be extremely pleasurable and sometimes extremely painful, scary and confusing. People on the autism spectrum are courageous and heroic, as every day they can face a multitude of feelings and emotions that most neuro-typical people would have difficulty coping with.

> We autistics wonder at non-autistic people and their acceptance of noise, lack of concentration and mercurial behaviour. When out in the world our experience is like being on a white knuckle ride being thrown unexpectedly from one fright to another. (Maguire, 2014, p.107)

We have worked with many children and young adults on the autism spectrum over many years. All of them were wonderfully different from each other, with immense variances in their characters and personalities, and all so intriguing to be around. We have learned a great deal about ourselves and others. Our interactions have allowed us to experience things differently and catch glimpses of a world that would be otherwise closed to us.

One of the areas that we have always focused on is the importance of play. Play is a fundamental area of learning and development and forms a basis for communication skills later in life. Play, however, does not always come naturally to children with autism, but this can be addressed within our work when using Building Language Using LEGO® Bricks.

Autism and play

> ...if the play is organized by grown-ups on the children's terms, the children find a common platform where – through play – they can gain social experiences, which otherwise can be difficult to learn. (Gammeltoft and Nordenhof, 2007, p.10)

There have been many studies, papers and books stating that the ability to play is fundamental to children's development. From Vygotsky's theory of cognition written in 1930 (reprinted 1978) to present-day publications (Lillard *et al.*, 2013), the evidence is substantial. For a normally developing child, play skills are present intuitively and can be seen clearly shortly after birth. A baby can recognize her mother's face at six weeks old and smile and at eight weeks may engage in a peek-a-boo game (BBC Health, 2013).

For children with autism, these skills are not instinctive and may not come naturally. Some developmental milestones achieved in typically developing children may be inaccessible to those on the autism spectrum without successful tuition. There are many interventions that target the teaching of specific skills to those on the spectrum; Building Language Using LEGO® Bricks is just one of them. It can provide a base for teaching a wide range of skills in a very appealing way.

There is growing evidence (Matson, Matson and Rivet, 2007) that shows conventional social skills methods may not always have the desired effect in supporting people with autism to overcome their social deficits. These studies now point to the benefits of more functional ways of teaching social skills that are delivered with contextual meaning and therefore potentially transferable into other areas (Jordan and Powell, 1995; Vermeulen, 2001). Again, Building Language Using LEGO® Bricks fits this model and we have seen skills transferred from our sessions into the classroom and playground.

What is language impairment?

The changes in the DSM-5 also saw changes in the classification of communication disorders, which now include:

- Language Disorder

- Speech Sound Disorder

- Childhood-onset Fluency Disorder

- Social (Pragmatic) Communication Disorder

- Unspecified Communication Disorder.

Consult the DSM-5 for definitions of each communication disorder.

The new clinical diagnosis of Social (Pragmatic) Communication Disorder (S(P)CD) describes social communication deficits that also form one component of the criteria for ASD. The DSM-5 clearly describes the differences between Social (Pragmatic) Communication Disorder and ASD (American Psychiatric Association, 2013).

In an article in the January 2016 issue of the *Bulletin* (the official magazine of the Royal College of Speech and Language Therapists), Professor Norbury (2016) lists the four key symptoms required for diagnosis of S(P)CD. These are difficulties in the following areas.

- Using language for social purposes, such as greeting and sharing information.

- Changing language and/or communication according to the social context or the needs of the listener.

- Following rules of discourse and narrative, e.g. turn taking, topic maintenance and using non-verbal communication cues to regulate conversation.

- Going beyond what is explicitly stated to make inferences or understand figurative language forms.

(Norbury, 2016)

Although the DSM-5 criteria for ASD and S(P)CD are somewhat controversial, when the social communication deficits are broken down into these four areas it can be seen how Building Language Using LEGO® Bricks may have a place in developing skills in all these areas.

Most children who present with any difficulties of communication are now referred to as having Speech, Language and Communication Needs (SLCN). This umbrella term encompasses all aspects of communication, that is: the ability to understand spoken language and to be able to generate spoken language to an age appropriate level, the ability to develop clear speech to an age appropriate level and the ability to communicate in socially appropriate ways to an age appropriate level.

Building Language Using LEGO® Bricks can address the majority of these communication skills, with the exception of developing clear speech. For advice on speech sound delay or disorders the reader is advised to contact their local speech and language therapy service.

Building Language Using LEGO® Bricks can facilitate the development of receptive and expressive language. In order to examine what we mean by 'language' it is helpful to refer to a model developed by Bloom and Lahey (1978). Bloom and Lahey define language as the knowledge of how to represent the world through a code of arbitrary signals.

Bloom and Lahey identify three connected types of knowledge: 'content', 'form' and 'use', each of which need to be well developed and coordinated for understanding, expression and successful communication.

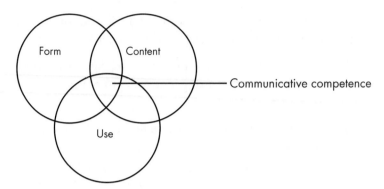

Figure 1.1: Bloom and Lahey's model of communication

Content is the speaker's knowledge of the world and is reflected through words and concepts.

Form is how the language is constructed. That is, the rules that govern how speech sounds combine to form words and how words combine to form meaningful sentences. This includes word order, grammar and morphology (the smallest units of meaning, e.g. –s plural).

Use is the pragmatics of communication. This is the ability to use language in socially appropriate ways, including how to be sensitive to the audience and the situation you are speaking in.

Communicative competence is derived from the ability to integrate content, form and use in a variety of situations. It follows then, that if any one or more of these systems does not develop as it should, then SLCN will arise.

We must also consider two further aspects of communication.

- Receptive language, that is the ability to understand spoken language

- Expressive language, that is the ability to use spoken language to communicate.

To become 'good' communicators using language we must develop receptive and expressive form, content and use.

Content: We must be able to understand a wide range of words that represent objects and people in the world and how these interact with each other (receptive).

We must also be able to use a wide range of words to represent what we see, know, think and feel (expressive).

Form: We must be able to understand the difference between speech sounds so that we can discriminate words. We must be able to understand the subtle meaning that is carried by more and more complex grammatical structures (receptive).

We must be able to combine speech sounds in language-specific ways to form words and must be able to produce a wide range of grammatical structures to convey a variety of meanings (expressive).

Use: We must learn to 'read' verbal and non-verbal communication, so that we can judge a speaker's intended meaning. Only some communication is reliant on the actual words; other aspects of meaning, such as emotions, are conveyed through 'how' we speak.

We must learn the culturally bound social conventions for the environment that we are communicating in. We must learn the 'how' to communicate for a wide variety of different people and contexts. This will include skills like how to make eye contact, turn-taking routines, how close we should stand to someone and how to be polite (expressive).

We must then combine all of these skills to 'say' what we want to say. That is, to communicate our intended meaning. We must then constantly monitor the effects of our communication on those we are speaking to, to ensure that our intended meaning has been received. Only at this stage can we be said to have developed communicative competence.

As can be seen from the brief description above, the development of language is highly complex. It is the subtle combination of environmental stimulation and the cognitive skills that a child brings to the language learning process that determines how language development progresses.

Cognitive skills will include the following.

• Attention control: the ability to attend to the world around us and to spoken language in the environment, so that we can connect the two.

- Memory: the ability to store words in our memory in an organized way so that we can retrieve them at a later date. Also the ability to store information about the world around us so that we can use this to help us communicate.

- Auditory perception: that is the brain's ability to discriminate between different speech sounds and words and then match them to meaning or its ability to hear only part of a word (maybe because of background noise) and to fill in the missing part so that you can still understand what is being said.

- Symbolic development: the ability to understand that one object can represent another or an idea. This is a vital developmental stage for language development, as language is the ultimate system of arbitrary symbols (words) that represent what we see, hear, think and feel. This can be seen in early childhood through play: a doll represents a baby; a cardboard box can become a boat.

- For complex activities like communication the brain has developed what is referred to as an executive system, which basically integrates all of these skills to allow us to set goals, coordinate complex activities (like communication) and use a constant feedback loop, so that we can judge how we are doing and adapt our communication accordingly.

Language impairment is a term that covers a range of difficulties in any or all of the areas discussed above. Only thorough unpicking of a child's skills and needs can reveal where in the language and cognitive system difficulties may lie. Once we can identify this, we can then plan intervention appropriately to ensure it is as effective and efficient as possible.

These impairments can be seen in children with a wide range of diagnoses, including the various communication disorders and autistic spectrum disorder. Language impairments may also be apparent in those with attention deficit disorders or intellectual (cognitive) disabilities and acquired brain damage.

The impact of these will be illustrated as the book progresses.

Chapter 2

Building Language Using LEGO® Bricks and LEGO® Therapy

Dr LeGoff (2004), targeted young people on the autism spectrum with an IQ of over 70. The cohort also had adequate language skills to allow them to participate in the sessions without the need for language facilitation.

Participants worked together to construct a model using LEGO® bricks, with the task being divided into three roles.

- The engineer, who interprets the instructions and communicates these to the other roles.

- The supplier, who selects the correct bricks (as directed by the engineer) and passes them to the builder.

- The builder, who places the bricks in the correct location on the model according to the engineer's directions.

Dr LeGoff states that due to the intrinsically motivating nature of building using LEGO® bricks, there is no need to use external reinforcers when using his approach. This is in keeping with recommendations by Attwood (1998) and Koegel, Singh and Koegel (2010) both of which advocate using a child's natural interests to motivate success with social communication.

It is worth noting that external reinforcers can be a good tool for some hard-to-reach students. This will be discussed in more detail throughout the book.

Building Language Using LEGO® Bricks

Building Language Using LEGO® Bricks is a flexible intervention derived from the original papers written in 2004 and 2008, but significantly adapted to meet the needs of children with severe receptive and expressive language disorders, including those on the autism spectrum.

Building Language Using LEGO® Bricks has been used as a successful tool to facilitate the development of receptive and expressive language and social communication skills within special and mainstream schools.

In the same way as described in LeGoff's paper in 2004, Building Language Using LEGO® Bricks uses LEGO® bricks as a medium for a division of labour task, with the end product being the constructed model. In both Building Language Using LEGO® Bricks and LeGoff's original approach, participants are assigned specific roles and have to work together to achieve the end goal (the constructed model).

It is not until you actually experience Building Language Using LEGO® Bricks first hand, that you realize just how much receptive and expressive language is needed to participate in what seems like a simple activity. Consider how difficult it would be to construct some flat-pack furniture without being able to see the instructions and only having someone tell you where to place and attach things. Then consider the same exercise, but you and your build partner both have learning disability, language impairment or autism. Maybe your partner has severe word-finding difficulties and they want to tell you to use the screwdriver but instead they tell you to use the hammer. A simple build may be fraught with frustrations and anger as communication breaks down.

We have worked with children with severe language disorders as well as those with autism. Due to the very nature of these diagnoses and the presenting needs of the young people we have adapted the sessions significantly; primarily by providing visual supports to aid language comprehension and use. During our Building Language Using LEGO® Bricks sessions, we have seen the children experience a range of emotions from joy and elation to anger and frustration. We guide them through these emotions and help them to problem solve and practise skills, which we hope will help them in their adult life.

Although we have seen changes in social communication skills (as described in the original research), the most significant outcome for the young people has been development in receptive and expressive language skills. Over a period of time we have learned from these successes (and our less successful sessions!) so that our practice has evolved into what we now refer to as Building Language Using LEGO® Bricks.

Some of the differences in the two therapeutic approaches can be seen clearly in Table 2.1. Each of these will be expanded in this chapter.

Table 2.1: Significant differences between LeGoff's approach and Building Language Using LEGO® Bricks

	LEGO® Therapy (described in the research paper: LeGoff, 2004)	Building Language Using LEGO® Bricks
Cognitive ability	IQ >70	Not specified
Age range	Below 14	No limit
Diagnosis	High Functioning Autism (HFA) and Asperger Syndrome (AS)	A variety of diagnoses included: autism (including Pathological Demand Avoidance (PDA)), specific language impairment, selective mutism, acquired brain injury, cerebral palsy (included Worster-Drought Syndrome), learning disability
Linguistic ability	Able to speak in phrases	Full range from verbal to non-verbal
Roles	Three roles: engineer supplier builder	Two roles: engineer (included supplier role) builder
Reinforcers	No external rewards	Tokens used

	LEGO® Therapy (described in the research paper: LeGoff, 2004)	Building Language Using LEGO® Bricks
Aims	Development of social communication skills: development of joint attention development of listening skills problem solving turn taking patience being part of a group eye contact (This is not a definitive list)	Development of: joint attention listening and attention control receptive and expressive language, particularly the number of information-carrying words that can be processed and used concept development (shape, colour, positional language, size and texture) problem solving turn taking patience eye contact (where appropriate) range of language functions, e.g. giving instructions, requesting, clarifying, communication repair increase self-esteem understanding self as part of a group. bilateral integration and fine motor skills

Cognitive abilities

Cognitive abilities in this context refers to the underlying non-verbal skills that allow children to learn, for instance, memory, visual and auditory perception, reasoning and problem-solving skills.

Building Language Using LEGO® Bricks has been used successfully with participants with a range of cognitive abilities, from HFA (no learning disability) to those with a diagnosis of complex learning difficulties.

26

Age range

This flexible intervention can be used with a range of participants regardless of age. Our experience has been with children and young people from 4 to 19. We have also trained people working in adult services.

Diagnosis

We have successfully run groups where partners have a variety of diagnoses and verbal skills. Criteria for selection of suitable build partnerships will be discussed in Chapter 5.

Linguistic ability

Building Language Using LEGO® Bricks can be adapted for use with a range of verbal abilities. Our experience has included children with high-level language skills to those with no verbal language, reliant on Alternative and Augmentative Communication strategies (AAC). Details of language and communication facilitation techniques will be expanded throughout the book. See Chapter 9 for an example of how to use Building Language Using LEGO® Bricks with a child who is reliant on AAC techniques to communicate with their build partner.

Roles

There are only two roles in the Building Language Using LEGO® Bricks approach. These are:

- the engineer, who interprets the instructions and communicates these to the builder

- the builder, who selects the correct bricks and places them in the designated location on the model, according to the engineer's directions.

On rare occasions we have reintroduced the third role of the 'supplier' to target a specific goal. For example, a colleague of ours successfully adapted Building Language Using LEGO® Bricks when working with a child with a total visual impairment. The child was given the supplier role, which enabled her to engage socially and feel part of the group from which she was often isolated. The bricks were organized into Brailled containers according to their colour. The supplier role allowed the child to participate meaningfully in the activity. This provided a safe and structured opportunity to begin to develop relationships with peers.

The children will experience both roles during a session.

To give the roles a clear definition, we introduced badges for the children to wear during the sessions (Appendix 10). We found this made it easier for the children to understand which role they were in and, more importantly, helped them with their transition into their second role. Badges for all three roles are included in Appendix 10 for those who may wish to include the supplier role.

Reinforcers

Part of the facilitator's role is to provide tokens throughout the sessions. The tokens can be a powerful visual aid to reinforce a variety of goals and achievements. These tokens do not form part of a token economy. Guidelines for their use will be expanded in Chapter 6.

We have provided a template for a simple paper token that can be used in Appendix 11, however, it is important that tokens are motivating and thus may need to be based around your child's specific interests. Parents have successfully used stickers or food rewards in place of tokens to reinforce targeted skills.

Chapter 3

Aims

Building Language Using LEGO® Bricks can be used to facilitate the development of a wide range of skills. The most significant of these are discussed in this chapter.

Development of joint attention

Joint attention is the ability to focus on the same stimuli as a communication partner. This is an important skill and is seen in early development. Joint attention is vital for many aspects of language development, particularly vocabulary learning and social skills development.

Michael Tomasello and Michael Jeffrey Farrar (1986) write about the importance of relatively extended episodes of joint attention focus between adult and child in providing non-linguistic scaffolding for the young child's early linguistic interactions (social skills).

The same authors also suggest that joint attention is vital for vocabulary development, presumably because such episodes are periods when the child is attentive, motivated and best able to determine the meaning of a communication partner's language. Lack of joint attention is an impairment often seen in autism and should be a target for early intervention.

Building Language Using LEGO® Bricks demands joint attention throughout the entire activity. Without it the end product (the constructed model) is not achieved.

Listening and attention control

A child needs good attention and listening skills to remember what has been said. They are then more likely to understand and respond appropriately. Good attention and listening skills are needed so that a child can:

- develop early social interactions with adults and other children

- understand words and follow instructions accurately

- develop vocabulary

- develop grammar, e.g. –ed for past tense, –s for plural

- develop accurate speech sounds, which leads on to phonic awareness and literacy development

- participate in conversations and class discussions and make friends

- develop incidental learning from the world around them

- understand when to respond in a social interaction.

Levels of listening and attention skills are therefore highly correlated to language development and academic achievement.

Table 3.1 is adapted from information by Cooper, Moodley and Reynell (1978). It is still very relevant and widely used in clinical practice.

Table 3.1: Developmental levels of attention control

Attention level	Effect on language	Strategies to help
Level 1: 0–1 year Child very distractible Attention fleeting	Child cannot attend to what you say	Discover child's motivators and incorporate into their preferred activity
Level 2: 1–2 years Child can attend to own choice of activity for a longer period of time but cuts self off from everything else	Your speech interferes with the activity child is doing Child needs to ignore you to concentrate	Give child time to complete own choice of activity Gain child's attention by calling their name and/or touching them
Level 3: 2–3 years Still single channelled attention but begins to attend to adults	Child can listen if he stops activity and looks at adult Needs adult prompts to do this	Call child's name before speaking, adult should join in child's preferred activity and relate language to this
Level 4: 3–4 years Single channelled but more easily controlled	Child looks automatically when adult speaks Can shift attention from task to speaker	Tell child it's time to listen Tell them that they can carry on working whilst listening to you – practise skill using an activity they can do with ease like colouring
Level 5: 4–5 years Integrated attention for short periods of time	Child no longer needs to look up when adult speaks Can listen at the same time as working or playing	Praise for good listening
Level 6: 5–6 years Integrated attention well established	Child listens and attends well in class	

In Building Language Using LEGO® Bricks attention and listening skills are targeted through the highly motivational nature of the activity. Tokens are used to reinforce longer and longer periods where a child will wait for a build partner's response.

Receptive and expressive language

The two key areas of language that appear to be influenced by Building Language Using LEGO® Bricks are:

- the number of information-carrying words understood and used

- development of early concepts.

These will be discussed below.

Information-carrying words (ICW)

(ICW are sometimes referred to as keywords.)

Knowles and Masidlover (1982) first introduced the concept of the *information-carrying word* in the Derbyshire Language Scheme. The concept looks at the pressure that spoken utterances place on auditory memory (a form of working memory). This form of memory is often impaired in children and adults with language impairment, learning difficulties and dyslexia.

An ICW is a word that carries meaning. It must be understood in order to comprehend accurately what has been said. Much of spoken language is redundant, for example the ability to follow the instruction 'put the circle in the box' is dependent on context, that is, the demands on the child's auditory (working) memory will change according to the context of the instruction.

EXAMPLE OF 0 ICW

'Put the circle in the box.'

If the child is last to take a turn, and there is only one shape left, they can follow the example of their peers and complete the activity without having to understand or remember any words in the spoken command (0 ICW). The need to understand 'in the box' becomes redundant by there being only one receptacle to place the shape in and by the example of classmates.

EXAMPLE OF 1 ICW

'Put the circle in the box.'

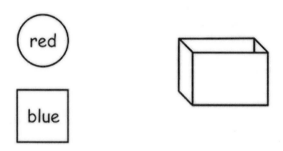

Figure 3.1: Context for 1 ICW

If there were two shapes left (circle and square), the child would have to understand the name of the shape 'circle' (as opposed to square) in order to select the correct shape. In this context the instruction becomes a 1 ICW command. The need to understand 'in the box' becomes redundant by there being only one receptacle to place the shape in and by the example of classmates.

EXAMPLE OF 2 ICW

'Put the red circle in the box.'

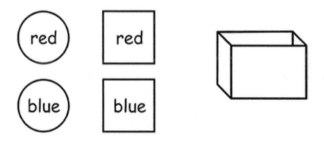

Figure 3.2: Context for 2 ICW

If the child must choose from a blue circle and a blue square *and* a red circle and a red square, they have to hold both the word for the shape and for the colour in their working memory. This is then a 2 ICW command.

EXAMPLE OF 3 ICW

'Put the red circle in the box.'

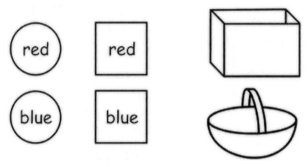

Figure 3.3: Context for 3 ICW

If the child must choose from a blue circle, a blue square, a red circle and a red square, and if there was also a choice of receptacle, for example a box and a basket, then the child must understand the colour, shape and receptacle name and hold this in their working memory in order to understand this command. This is then a 3 ICW command.

Building Language Using LEGO® Bricks challenges the number of ICW understood and used. The number of ICW can gradually be increased as the participant's skills develop. Strategies to increase and decrease the number of ICW will be discussed in later chapters.

In typical language development, as a rough guide, a child of two years should understand 2 ICW, at three years they should understand 3 ICW and at four years they should understand 4 ICW.

Development of early concepts

Basic concepts are ideas that help us represent tangible and less tangible aspects of our world within our memory (often referred to as semantic memory). They help us to understand the relationship between things within it. Labels (words) can then be assigned to these concepts to help us represent them in our internal thought processes and to express them to others.

Basic concepts needed for success in school can be divided into categories.

- Colours, e.g. red, blue, pink, brown.

- Quantities, e.g. more, less, few, many, some, least.

- Directions, e.g. around, through, open, close.

- Sequences, e.g. first, next, before, after, finally, now.

- Size, e.g. big, small, huge, tiny.

- Shapes, e.g. circle, square, oval, diamond.

- Textures, e.g. smooth, rough, blunt, sharp, hard, soft.

- Time, e.g. day, week, month, year, morning, afternoon, evening, late, early.

- Positional, e.g. in, on, under, next to, behind, above, below, between, opposite, end, corner.

- Descriptions, e.g. empty, full, loud, quiet, young, old.

- Social/emotional, e.g. happy, sad, angry, frightened, surprised, worried.

Positional language and social/emotional are particular issues for children with autism.

Early concept development is strongly linked to academic success (Breen, 1984). Gardner (1991) stresses the importance of word and concept knowledge for academic achievement, literacy and lifelong learning. Concepts help us to represent complex ideas as language in our thoughts. They therefore help us with the process of higher level thinking skills like problem solving, inference and deduction.

To progress in the education system even children at preschool level need to be able to understand many of the labels (words) that we use to represent these concepts. Take the following for example: '*First* go and wash your hands. *Then* get your lunchbox. It's *behind* the *big, red* cupboard.'

Understanding of basic concepts is vital to success in many curriculum areas, particularly maths and science. The education system within the UK recognizes the importance of understanding these concepts and many good preschool and reception teachers will specifically teach them. However, due to the less tangible and changing nature of these concepts, children with language impairments or autism or those with learning difficulties will find them more difficult to understand and will need additional help.

Consider the concept of 'big'. This changes according to context. A big mouse will always be much smaller than a small elephant. The concept of 'yesterday' changes too. If today is Tuesday then yesterday was Monday, but tomorrow yesterday will be Tuesday (today)! It is no wonder these concepts are so hard to learn.

Learning to label emotions

In order to label an emotional state, we first have to experience the emotion. We need to recognize the 'symptoms' of this emotion in our own bodies. We may all feel emotions in different ways. Take 'anxiety' for instance. Some may feel 'butterflies in the tummy'; some may feel a tightening across the chest or a stiffening of the shoulders. How we experience the emotion does not matter. What is important is that we can recognize this emotion and can then match this to a spoken label of 'anxious' or 'nervous'.

It can be difficult to evoke emotions in children in order to label them in a classroom or home setting. Often the routine and security of these settings result in passivity or neutral emotions.

Building Language Using LEGO® Bricks can be used to evoke emotion in a manageable way. For some, waiting for a build partner to respond can provoke increased frustration or anxiety. This can then be highlighted, labelled and controlled.

The first step in learning strategies to control our emotions is to identify them.

The facilitator can gradually increase the demand on a child so they can experience enough of an emotion to help identify and label it without it leading to a total meltdown. To do this the facilitator will have to have good knowledge of the child. For this reason, this target is best worked on during the later stages of the intervention.

Problem solving and communication repair

Communication breakdown occurs when the message you are trying to convey has not been understood as you had intended. The issue may be with the speaker, the listener or environmental factors. Communication breakdown is a feature of typical communication and happens to us all. It is how we repair the breakdown that demonstrates our skill as a communicator. This process is complex and involves the following stages.

- Identify the breakdown: Something has gone wrong!

- Identify what has gone wrong: Was it me or them? Is it too noisy and they didn't hear me? Did I use the wrong word? Did I speak too fast? Were they listening to me?

- Choosing a repair strategy: How can I make it better (taking into account the listener and the environment)?

- Formulate and implement the repair strategy: Say it again, say their name to gain their attention, use a different word etc.

- Learn from my successes to help me communicate more successfully in the future.

Children with autism and those with language impairments will experience breakdown in communication more frequently than most. They may not recognize that communication has broken down and will assume the listener has understood them. They will often also lack the skills to repair the breakdown without help.

Developing socially acceptable ways of repairing communication breakdown is fundamental in being accepted in society. An example of this in a Building Language Using LEGO® Bricks session follows.

> If I asked you to pick up a blue brick and you picked up a red one, my attempt to repair this could make or break our relationship. Compare: 'No stupid, I said the red one!' with: 'Sorry, I'll say it again: red.'

This skill is frequently challenged and practised in Building Language Using LEGO® Bricks sessions. The role of the facilitator is vital in developing this skill. Work on this process is discussed in Chapter 6. Resource prompts are included in Appendix 9.

Turn taking and patience

Deficits in turn taking are common in autism and can be a feature of language impairment for some. Turn taking is a vital, early-developing skill. It forms an essential building block for many higher level abilities.

The division of labour to achieve a joint goal is at the core of Building Language Using LEGO® Bricks and naturally facilitates turn taking in a highly motivating way.

Participants will have to learn to wait their turn if they are to achieve the end goal. The facilitator's role in this will be expanded in Chapter 6 and strategies will be discussed in the case studies in Chapter 9.

Range of language functions

Many functions of language are challenged in a structured way during Building Language Using LEGO® Bricks sessions. These include directing, questioning, repairing, confirming and following direction. Our experience has been that this intervention is particularly powerful in developing skills in repairing communication breakdown; that is, the ability to correct people in a socially appropriate way when they have not understood you.

A list of communication functions targeted by this approach can be found in Chapter 8. This list can be used to establish a baseline for intervention, to set targets and to measure progress.

Bilateral integration and fine motor skills

Fine motor skills are the skills that use the smaller muscles of the hands, for example when we fasten buttons, use scissors or pencils or manipulate building bricks. Difficulties in the development of fine motor skills impact upon developing independence and academic success.

The building blocks necessary to develop fine motor skills include developing bilateral integration and the ability to cross the midline.

Bilateral integration means the ability to use both hands together with one hand leading, for example when you open a jar lid using the other hand to stabilize the jar, or when you add a brick to a build using the non-dominant hand to stabilize the structure.

Crossing the midline is the ability to cross an imaginary line that runs down a person's body from their nose to their pelvis, dividing the body into two halves. Children who do not cross the midline tend to pick up things placed on the right with their right hand and things placed on their left with their left hand. It is important that the child develops the ability to cross the midline as this helps the two halves of the brain to communicate with each other. The cortex of the brain is also divided into two halves (hemispheres). These two halves usually have responsibility for different skills. Generally speaking, language skills are predominantly based in the left hemisphere and spatial skills in the right. It is important that these two hemispheres communicate so that tasks requiring a range of skills can develop smoothly.

When constructing a model, children are required to use both hands together, providing vital practice of these skills through the use of a very motivating activity.

We have worked closely with our occupational therapy colleagues when developing Building Language Using LEGO® Bricks and have seen a clear progression of skills in this area.

Some children have required use of the larger bricks (DUPLO®) in the initial stages of the intervention. We have then gradually reduced the size of the bricks or altered the complexity of the build to increase the physical challenge.

If the child you are working with presents with fine motor control difficulties, we would strongly recommend seeking the advice of an occupational therapist.

Eye contact

It can be beneficial to prompt those children who do not have a diagnosis of autism to look towards the person that they are engaging with. This promotes good social skills and can help with interaction. This should be done with caution though, as it may be that the child is using all of their concentration on formulating a sentence and cannot do this while looking directly at their partner (see information on development of attention control).

For those with autism, eye contact should never be forced. Many people with autism are hypersensitive to visual stimuli and eye contact is not only uncomfortable, but can also be unbearably painful.

We also have to bear in mind that some people with autism have sensory processing difficulties and may not be able to engage verbally if they are engaging visually. This inability to 'switch channels' can be seen in the autistic child in many classrooms. Pupils on the spectrum are often asked to 'look at the teacher' when in fact they may be fully engaged in the lesson using their auditory channel, as this is the one that is most helpful at the time.

In Building Language Using LEGO® Bricks we encourage build partners to use each other's names to gain attention. We may prompt them by asking them to look up towards their partner and find a place to look at that feels comfortable. This may be their partner's chin, forehead or shoulder area. Tokens can be used to reinforce this so that it becomes a more natural reaction.

Chapter 4

Why Building Language Using LEGO® Bricks Works

There are many reasons why we believe this intervention is effective. The activity itself is not age or gender specific. In fact, it is universally accepted that you can be 9 months or 99 years old and 'play' with LEGO® bricks. It can be a solitary activity or something to enjoy with friends or family. By using LEGO® bricks as an intervention to encourage language and communication, we feel that we are already winning a sometimes difficult battle. In an article about using LEGO® bricks therapeutically, Uta Frith (Emeritus Professor of Cognitive Development at University College London) describes the motivating sensory elements of LEGO® bricks in the way they look, sound and feel (2012).

When we look at the theories around autism we can see why Building Language Using LEGO® Bricks can tap into areas that can be difficult to reach.

Below are some of the psychological theories on the nature of autism. They are brief, simplistic snapshots of the theories in relation to Building Language Using LEGO® Bricks and are not complete in their explanations. These theories are highly complex. This book is not the forum to provide definitions for them in their full context.

Theory of mind

Theory of mind is a term used to describe self-awareness and awareness of others. It is an understanding that other people have intentions, desires and beliefs that are different to your own (Baron-Cohen, Leslie and Frith, 1985).

This is an area that can cause great frustration to those on the autism spectrum and their parents, carers, teachers and support staff. Some children are extremely rigid in their thinking and find it very difficult to accept another point of view. We have found that with this intervention we can introduce theory of mind in a very basic and naturalistic way. Even something as simple as deciding who is going to be the builder or engineer first is an initial step in the art of compromising and the start of understanding other people's desires.

During initial sessions, build partners are seated on the same side of the table, so that positional language concepts can be developed. To introduce basic understanding of theory of mind, we would place the children opposite one another. They then have to consider their build partner's perspective in order for the build to be successful. To understand, 'Put the red brick *behind* the blue one,' the child has to consider that what is *behind* to them will be *in front of* to a build partner on the opposite side of the table. This can sometimes take moving of chairs in order to experience the different perspectives.

Weak central coherence

Frith (2003, p.134) describes weak central coherence as: 'the unusual ability to disregard context'.

For many people on the autism spectrum this can be the case. It can be very difficult to see something as a whole, as it is the tiny details that catch the child's attention.

Typically developing children will retain a general impression of a situation. They will use the details to gain an overall picture. Those with weak central coherence will not be able to piece together detail to form a whole. They will see the individual trees but not the forest.

Although the lack of central coherence can be very strong, an intervention like Building Language Using LEGO® Bricks may help some to see the 'bigger picture' or 'get the gist' by its very nature of building, where all of the small pieces fit together to make a larger model.

Executive functions

Boucher (2009, p.170) describes executive functions as: 'the set of cognitive processes that are involved in the organisation and control of mental and physical activity'.

It is executive functions that enable us to switch from one activity to another or stop altogether and start on something else. It is also the ability to predict the behaviour of others. The cognitive thought process for this involves a great deal of flexibility of thinking, which can be difficult for some individuals on the autism spectrum.

Building Language Using LEGO® Bricks can help with planning, organizing and problem solving and therefore with the area of executive functioning. We feel that the task of building a model with a partner 'forces' the participants to engage their skills of executive functions in a structured but naturalistic way.

Take, for example, the difficulty that people on the autism spectrum may have in stopping an incomplete task. We have found that 99 per cent of the children that we have worked with have overcome this within Building Language Using LEGO® Bricks sessions.

You will see in Chapter 6 the process for facilitating this acceptance.

- We took photographs of the models that were 'mid-build'.

- We placed the build in a locked cupboard until the next session.

- The children were also given a photograph of their model so they could match it when the build started again. Initially we were asked many times by the children to see their model, which we always complied with, so that they knew it was how they had left it.

By following this procedure consistently we found that it wasn't too long before the children trusted us. This enabled them to progress onto a more complex model built over a longer period of time (several sessions). They learned to stop the build when it was incomplete without experiencing feelings of stress and anxiety, knowing that it would continue again from the point they had left it.

Poor ability to jointly attend

We have noticed many times that some of the children only needed to see the finished photograph of the model for a split second and they were able to recreate it perfectly without the need for the instructions. This negated the need for any social interaction with their build partner. For this reason we introduced a small screen to conceal the photos or instructions and establish joint attention from the very start of the sessions.

Theories of word learning

The nature of vocabulary learning and acquisition is very complex. Much research has been dedicated to this subject over the years. We now have a much clearer idea of which word elements we need to learn as well as how we learn a word.

It has been estimated widely that the average adult has 30,000 words in their vocabulary (Clark, 1995). To get to this point a child has to learn an average of six to eight new words every day throughout their school years.

A child learns a spoken word through listening to spoken language, picking out which combination of sounds represent which objects and attaching meaning to them. In order to do this, they must experience exposure to the objects in their environment so that they can learn about them through their senses. Let's look at the example of learning the word 'cat'. The child will handle the cat and so learn it is soft and fluffy. It hears it and learns that it makes a specific set of sounds. It sees it and learns it has four legs and is a certain colour. All this information is called semantic knowledge. Semantic knowledge builds slowly with more exposures to the word in different contexts. So a child may encounter a different cat and realize that they come in a range of colours and patterns. They may learn (painfully) that cats have claws and use them if you pull their tails! Children then begin to build more and more refined semantic understanding of a word. They refine this further through exclusion. They may see a dog and say 'cat'; the adult will then correct them and label the new creature a dog. This exclusion refines the child's understanding further. This process of gradual refinement through experience in different contexts is called mapping. Mapping helps the child to build organized associations between words in their growing lexicon. So they will learn a cat is an animal, it is part of a sub group called pets and is associated with words like purr, stroke, fur, claws and tail. Research has found that a child needs at least 12 mapping exposures to a word in different contexts to gain a full understanding of that word (Stahl and Nagy, 2005).

Building Language Using LEGO® Bricks helps with word learning, particularly the learning of concepts, as it provides numerous (mapping) exposures to concept words within slightly different but controllable exposures. It is the facilitator's role, within sessions, to control the context of these exposures to ensure a gradual building of concept knowledge (see Chapter 6).

It is useful to think of the learning of vocabulary as compiling a filing cabinet full of words in your memory. For each word there will be sub divisions within the file for different elements of the word. Semantic knowledge as discussed above is one of these files. Others include: phonological knowledge, syntactic knowledge and orthographic knowledge (for those words we are able to read).

Phonological knowledge is the speech sound make up of a word, for instance, what sound does it begin and end with, what words does it rhyme with and how many syllables make up the word? These are the sort of things that we often recall during 'tip of the tongue' experiences. When we know a word but can't quite retrieve it, we often are able to say, 'It's a short word and it begins with ...'

Syntactic knowledge is knowledge of the rules that govern how you combine the word with others to form a sentence. It builds from hearing words used within a variety of sentences. Through this process children 'pick up' what category a word belongs to, so they will understand that cat is a noun. They will of course not know the term noun but will understand that you can add /s/ to make the word plural 'cats', but do not say 'cating'.

Building Language Using LEGO® Bricks can help build this knowledge by exposing the child to subtly varied sentences containing the target concept. 'Put the red brick *behind* the blue one.' 'Put the green rectangle *behind* the yellow one.'

Orthographic knowledge is stored memory of how the word looks when it is written down. That is, your ability to recognize and read the word. This can be facilitated during sessions through consistent association of the written word and symbol with the concept in varying contexts.

In conclusion, Building Language Using LEGO® Bricks can facilitate all these aspects of word knowledge by concentrating exposures to the targeted word in subtly varied contexts. It works on helping the child build up semantic knowledge and then helps them to know how the word can be used within connected speech. The repetitive nature of the builds allows mapping exposures to concepts in far greater concentration than would usually be experienced. This, then, speeds the natural process of word learning.

Chapter 5

Starting Off

Pairing clients

Choosing the right partners is essential to the success of this intervention. We have learned through experience that it is immediately obvious if the partnership is not going to work! We have found it useful to consider the following criteria when selecting build partners.

- Language skills: Partners do not have to share the same level of skill. Some of the most successful partnerships can involve one child with high-level language skills and one with very little expressive language. The selection will be determined more by the targets you wish to achieve, e.g. developing patience, empathy and communication repair strategies with a less linguistically able peer (see case examples in Chapter 9).

- Cognitive skills: Most of our successful partnerships have shared a similar level of cognitive ability. We have found that large differences in cognitive ability can lead to frustration and relationship breakdown.

- Personality and relationships: Understanding and knowing the children we have worked with has informed our selection. For readers working in a new environment we would recommend a short playground observation (where possible) or use a session to engage in an activity to assess suitability for partnerships. We would suggest that this activity would not include play using LEGO® bricks.

The advice of others who know the children well should always be taken into consideration.

- Targets: Selecting children to achieve specific targets will influence partnerships. We have paired children because they have shared high levels of anxiety and thus have used Building Language Using LEGO® Bricks sessions to develop self-esteem through high levels of achievement. We have also partnered children to challenge their concept development or the number of information-carrying words they can use or understand. The case studies, later in the book, will cover a range of targets. Targets will often develop and change through the course of a block of sessions.

Assessment – establishing a baseline of skills

It is important with any therapeutic intervention that we establish what the child is already capable of. This way we can ensure that our intervention sets just the right level of challenge to develop skills without being unachievable. It also gives us a way of measuring how much progress has been made or how effective the intervention has been (outcome measure).

This chapter will describe a series of informal test activities that can be used to establish skill levels in the key language areas that are challenged by Building Language Using LEGO® Bricks, namely:

- understanding and use of concepts (shape, size, position and colour)
- the number of information-carrying words (ICW) that are understood and used.

We also cover the 'pitfalls' in assessing language skills, and try to offer some guidance to overcome these as much as possible.

What am I testing?

The key to any successful test is to know what you are assessing. This may sound an obvious statement but all tests may 'tap into' a number of skills, so it is vital that you know which of these skills are being reflected in the results.

All the tests described below rely on the person being tested (the child) listening to an instruction and then making a choice (by pointing or by performing an action). Vital to this process is an ability to scan all options visually before making their choice. It is necessary to establish the ability to see and scan visually all the options available. Without this ability the test results may not reflect language skills but may tell you more about visual organization skills.

Most of us scan visually from left to right, starting at the top and scanning from left to right gradually working towards the bottom. If visual scanning is an issue, teaching to scan in this organized fashion may be necessary. This skill is a vital prerequisite to reading. Note that in some cultures and languages scanning may be from right to left or vertical.

If you find that scanning a large selection of items is an issue, you can reduce the impact on your test results in two ways.

- Reduce the number of options offered, where possible, to a minimum of four and arrange them in a single horizontal line.

- Physically draw attention to each option and ensure the child looks at each option prior to giving the test language stimuli.

Many of the test procedures below rely upon the child 'pointing to' an item to indicate their response to a spoken word or phrase. Recognition of the meaning conveyed by pointing is reliant upon an ability to jointly attend to an object. This is a well-documented difficulty for some children with autism. If the child has poor language skills, then eye pointing should be taken as an indicator rather than pointing with a finger. If visual scanning is known to be an issue for the child you are working with, it may be necessary to demonstrate the required response through several trials before carrying out the test proper. This will ensure that the results are a true reflection of language comprehension.

Tests should be designed only to test one concept or language structure at a time. The informal test activities below have been designed to follow this principle. It is essential, then, that the choice of materials and the language used are adhered to exactly as described. Without this strict adherence to test instructions you may not be testing the language skills you think you are testing.

Testing understanding of colour names

All colours used in this test should be presented in the same 'nameless' shape so that the only changeable concept is the actual colour. This will avoid confusion and make it more obvious to the child what is being asked for.

Some colours have been included in Appendix 3, however blank templates are also included for you to test colours relevant to whatever bricks you are working with.

It is vital to bear in mind visual scanning skills as described above. This will determine how many colour choices you offer at one time and how these should be arranged on the table.

Test procedure

Equipment

- Coloured picture cards are provided in Appendix 3. These should be copied onto card and cut up so that items can be selected and placed in front of the child.

Procedure

1. Place a number of colour pictures on the table in front of the child.

2. Ask them to 'show me [name a colour]', e.g. 'show me yellow'.

    It may be necessary to practise this process several times before you start the test proper so the child is sure about the pointing response that is required.

Always use the same language structure 'show me...'. This way the 'show me...' part of the instruction becomes redundant so that only the colour name is tested. Alternatively, if the child is used to assessments, with a little demonstration you may be able just to say the colour name to elicit a response.

3. Use the checklist included in Appendix 1 to note which colour names are correctly identified.

It is not necessary to test every colour individually. It may be good to test some of the more common colours to establish a baseline and then make a note of those that appear to be a problem during a build activity. These can always be tested at a later date.

Testing understanding of prepositions (positional concepts)

Prepositions are words that describe the position of objects or people in relation to each other, for example, *in, on, under, between, in front of* and *behind*. In order to develop a good understanding of these concepts, a child must have reasonably developed body awareness, so they can judge where their body is in space. Children who present with difficulties in this area often find it hard to learn prepositions as they may find it hard to judge where things are in relation to themselves or other objects.

Building Language Using LEGO® Bricks constantly challenges the understanding of prepositions through the use of a motivating build activity. It can therefore be a really powerful way to develop understanding of these vital positional concepts.

There is a clear developmental order to the acquisition of positional language. Table 5.1 is taken from the work of Wiig and Semelp and depicts the ages of acquisition of some of the commonly used prepositions.

Table 5.1: Development of prepositions

Type	Preposition	Age of acquisition
Locative	In	2.0 to 2.6 years
Locative	On	2.6 to 3.0 years
Locative	Under	2.6 to 3.0 years
Directional	Off	2.0 to 2.6 years
Directional	Out of	2.6 to 3 years
Directional	Away from	2.6 to 3 years
Directional	Towards	3.0 to 3.6 years
Directional	Up	3.0 to 3.6 years
Directional	Down	4.6 to 5.0 years
Locative	In front of	3.6 to 4.0 years
Locative	In back of	3.6 to 4.0 years
Locative	Next to	3.6 to 4.0 years
Locative	Beside	4.0 to 4.6 years
Directional	Around	3.6 to 4.0 years
Locative	Ahead of	5.0 to 5.6 years
Locative	Behind	5.0 to 5.6 years

Some concepts are more difficult to learn than others because they are relative to the position of the subject. For example, the concept of 'on' or 'under' does not change depending upon your perspective. A person would be in the same position if they were standing 'on' a wall whichever side of the wall you were viewing them from. However, with the concept of 'in front of' or 'behind' a person's position will change depending on which side of the wall you are viewing from. These latter concepts are more difficult to learn and to teach as they are not static.

Generally speaking, children will learn positional concepts first in relation to their own bodies, for example they are 'in' the bath or 'under' the table or the ball is 'in front of' them. The developmental sequence is described below.

1. Learn the concept in relation to your own body (the ball is behind me).

2. Generalize these concepts to other people (what is behind Mum?).

3. Then to objects (what is next to the chair?). Remember for in front of and behind this would initially have to be an object with an obvious front and back.

4. Then recognize these concepts in pictures.

It is essential to have a good understanding of the concepts of 'front' and 'back' as a prerequisite to learning 'in front of' and 'behind'. Once this is established, it is best to teach the concept in relation to the child's own body and then to generalize it to an object with a definite front and back, like a chair or a car. You can then move on to the trickier task of teaching these concepts, with objects that depend upon perspective, for example 'stand *behind* the line'.

Building bricks don't usually have a definite front and back and thus present the most challenging level for some positional concepts. It may, therefore be necessary to sit participants next to each other on the same side of the table during Building Language Using LEGO® Bricks sessions targeting these concepts, so that they can share the same perspective. Once understanding is established you can then move participants to sit opposite each other to increase the challenge. They will then have to be aware of their partner's perspective on the build. This is a great way of working on the foundations of theory of mind.

Test procedure

It is important to ensure that the only variable during the test activity is the preposition being requested. To ensure this, it is necessary to provide the same coloured bricks for each test item and to use the same language structures to request a response.

Equipment

• Three red, rectangle bricks with eight dots.

Procedure

For most prepositions you will only need two bricks, however, to test understanding of the preposition 'between' you will need all three bricks.

1. Place one brick on the table in front of the child and hold the other brick in your hand.

2. Give the child the brick from your hand and say 'put it [name a preposition]', e.g. 'put it *on* the brick' or 'put it *behind* the brick'. As you give the command, point towards the brick on the table. It is essential that you only point towards the brick and do not touch it, as this could be confusing, e.g. a touch to the top of the brick may give a non-verbal clue to place the brick on top, whereas a touch to the side may non-verbally convey 'next to'.

3. Record the response on the assessment checklist in Appendix 1. Remove the bricks and set up for the next preposition.

4. To test 'between' it will be necessary to have two bricks on the table in front of the child with a small space between the bricks. Then follow the same procedure as above.

Remember to always use the same language structures. This will ensure that all language except the preposition word will become redundant by the repetitive activity.

Again, it is not necessary to test all positional concepts. Use the 'Development of prepositions' table (Table 5.1) to establish an order for testing. If the earlier concepts are not understood, it is unlikely that the later acquired ones will be known. This sequence can then be used as a guide for teaching. You could select build models that will challenge understanding of these earlier concepts and work towards understanding of the more mature concepts.

Testing understanding of shape

Children tend to learn the names of two dimensional (2D) shapes before they learn three dimensional (3D) shapes. The national curriculum in England, year 1 programme of study includes teaching children to recognize and label common 2D and 3D shapes.

Recognition of shape and comparison of shape properties is highly dependent upon well-developed visual perceptual skills. If this area appears to be a specific difficulty for the child you are working with, assessment of visual perceptual skills by a qualified occupational therapist may be indicated.

The use of 2D or 3D shape names during build activities will depend upon the emphasis of your teaching. If 2D names are not yet established it is often best to describe bricks according to these, for example a cube-shaped brick could be described as a square, with attention drawn to the shape of the top surface of the brick.

To test understanding of some of the common 2D shapes

Equipment

- Shape drawings in Appendix 4. Copy these onto card and cut into separate shapes so that you can present the number and layout of shape options according to the child's visual scanning skills.

Procedure

1. Place a number of shape cards in front of the child. A minimum of four in a horizontal line is best.

2. Draw the child's attention to the shapes and ensure they have visually scanned all options.

3. Say 'show me the [name a shape]', e.g. 'show me the *rectangle*'.

4. Mark the child's response on the assessment checklist in Appendix 1.

5. Remove the shapes and place four more options in front of the child.

Again, it is not necessary to assess all shapes but you may wish to assess some of those included in the build you are going to use.

We have not been able to include materials to assess 3D shapes, however these can be found on education resources websites. When assessing understanding of 3D shapes it is essential to remember the following principles.

- Only change one variable at a time, so ensure that all shapes you use are the same size and colour and only change the shape.

- Test understanding of 3D shape names with real objects before you use pictures of 3D shapes.

Testing concepts of measure

Many of the concepts used to describe size and measurement are relative, that is they are changeable depending upon the object being measured, for example a *big* mouse will always be much *smaller* than a *small* elephant. This makes these concepts difficult to learn and to test.

The tests described below are based on understanding of these concepts in relation to bricks, however, it is good to test in a number of ways in order to establish a solid baseline of skills.

As before, keep variables to a minimum, so use the same colour and type of brick where possible.

Test procedure

Equipment

- Same coloured bricks fitting the description of the size concepts to be tested, e.g. to test the concept 'big' you would need:

  - one red rectangle with six dots (3 x 2 dot arrangement).

  - one red rectangle with 12 dots (3 x 4 dot arrangement).

- It is vital that the big brick is both wider and longer than the first. If you presented a brick with a 10 x 2 dot arrangement this would represent the concept of *long*. A 3 x 3 dot arrangement would then become a square shape so would change a variable that should be static, i.e. shape (both bricks should be a rectangle).

- It is also essential to consider the depth of the brick. If you present one brick that is flat and one that is fat or deeper you have introduced another concept. This should only be introduced if testing the concepts of *flat* and *fat* or *deep* depending what you decide to name this concept.

Procedure

1. Place two bricks (demonstrating opposites of the concept you wish to test, e.g. big/little or long/short) in front of the child.

2. Make sure they have visually scanned all options.

3. Say, 'Which brick is [name the concept]?' e.g. 'Which brick is *long*?'

4. Record the response on the assessment checklist in Appendix 1.

5. Remove the bricks and present two more bricks to test the next concept.

As with all the tests, ensure you use the same language structures and practise the response so that all language apart from the concept name becomes redundant by repetition.

Testing the number of ICW understood

The concept of ICW is discussed in Chapter 3. To recap, an ICW is a word that must be understood in order to comprehend accurately what is being said. Much of spoken language is made redundant by context, repetition and non-verbal clues that accompany what we say. Many of the smaller grammatical words we use like 'the' or 'is/are' add only small detail to our understanding and so are not necessary to understanding the main 'gist' of what is being said. It is the ICW that add the essential content to our speech. It is vital then, when assessing understanding of spoken language, to measure how many of these key words can be processed in the same utterance.

The processing of ICW is dependent upon a child's auditory working memory capacity. That is the number of key words that can be held in working memory in order to process them for meaning.

An ICW is one where a choice has to be made in order to understand accurately the word. So, if I were to offer the reader just a red brick and to hold out my hand and command, 'give me the red brick' it is likely that you would be able to respond accurately to this command even if you did not understand the colour name 'red'. However, if I were to offer a red and a blue brick and give the same command, 'give me the red brick', the reader then has to choose between two different colours, so has to understand the word 'red' (see Chapter 3 for examples of ICW).

It follows then, that we can increase or decrease the number of ICW in a command by increasing or decreasing the choices we offer.

In the tests described below it is vital that the materials are presented exactly as described and that the stimulus language is strictly adhered to. This will ensure that the correct number of choices are offered for each ICW level.

As on all previous tests, it is essential that the child is able to scan all options visually before making a response. The number of bricks that must be scanned will increase with the number of ICW.

This test is reliant on an understanding of the concepts of shape, size, position and colour. If there have been any gaps in this knowledge, evidenced by previous test results, then this test will not be valid. Other assessments of ICW comprehension should be sought. Test procedures from the Derbyshire Language Scheme (Knowles and Madislover, 1982) are recommended.

We have tried to use those positional and size-related concepts that are known to develop first in this test procedure. The colours used in these tasks can be replaced by those you know the child understands, however, you must ensure that the correct number of 'choices' is preserved for each level.

Two activities are described for each level. Further activities can be added following the same principles but varying colour or shape concepts. It is important to carry out a number of trials so that you are sure that responses are due to accurate understanding and not chance.

1 ICW level

All of the tests described above that test shape, colour, size and positional concepts require understanding at a 1 ICW level. If the child has succeeded in a number of these tests, they have already demonstrated understanding at a 1 ICW level.

2 ICW level

Equipment

- One big, red brick.
- One small, red brick.

- One big, blue brick.
- One small, blue brick.

Procedure

Hold out your hand and say 'Give me the *big, red* brick.'

Equipment

- One red, square brick.
- One red, rectangle brick.
- One blue, square brick.
- One blue, rectangle brick.

Procedure

Hold out your hand and say 'Give me the *square blue* brick.'

3 ICW level

Equipment

- One big, blue, square brick.
- One small, blue, square brick.
- One big, red, square brick.
- One small, red, square brick.
- One big, red, rectangle brick.
- One small, red, rectangle brick.
- One big, blue, rectangle brick.
- One small, blue, rectangle brick.

Procedure

Hold out your hand and say 'Give me the *big, red, rectangle* brick'.

Equipment

- One big, blue, square brick.
- One small, blue, square brick.
- One big, red, square brick.
- One small, red, square brick.
- One big, white rectangle brick.

Procedure

1. Demonstrate taking a brick and placing it *under* the white brick.
2. Remove and replace that brick.
3. Demonstrate placing a different brick *on* the white brick.
4. Remove and replace that brick
5. Say, 'Put the *big, red* brick *under* this one' and point towards (but do not touch) the white brick.

Equipment

- One big, blue, square brick.
- One small, blue, square brick.
- One big, red, square brick.
- One small, red, square brick.
- One big, white rectangle brick.

Procedure

Say, 'Put the *small, blue* brick *on* this one' and point towards (but do not touch) the white brick.

4 ICW level

Equipment

- One big, blue, square brick.
- One small, blue, square brick.
- One big, red, square brick.
- One small, red, square brick.
- One big, red, rectangle brick.
- One small, red, rectangle brick.
- One big, blue, rectangle brick.
- One small, blue, rectangle brick.
- One big, white rectangle brick.

Procedure

1. Demonstrate taking a brick and placing it *under* the white brick.
2. Remove and replace that brick.
3. Demonstrate placing a different brick *on* the white brick.
4. Remove and replace that brick.
   Say, 'Put the *big, red, square* brick *under* this one' and point towards (but do not touch) the white brick.
   Replace all bricks.
   Say, 'Put the *big, blue, rectangle* brick *on* this one' and point towards (but do not touch) the white brick.

Record all responses on the assessment checklist in Appendix 1.

Chapter 6

Progressing Skills
The Role of the Facilitator

The adult who is helping to 'run' this intervention is referred to as 'the facilitator'. The Oxford dictionary defines a facilitator as: 'A person or thing that makes an action or process easy or easier.'

This definition is important as it underlines the fact that the adult is there to *help* the children with an activity rather than to *do* the activity for them. This notion is fundamental to the success of this intervention.

The role of the facilitator is vital to this intervention. The skill of the facilitator in moving children through small-step learning is the one factor that determines how successful this intervention will be. For that reason, we have set out this role in detail throughout this chapter.

The number of facilitators required per build partnership will vary with need. We have worked with children with complex needs and thus our experience has been that the intervention has initially been staff intensive.

The minimum staffing level has been one adult (facilitator) with each build partnership (two children). However, in the initial stages we have had many partnerships that required two facilitators (one for each participant). This can be useful when you are building your skills as a facilitator, as it is difficult to consider the targets and prompts required for two children at the same time. This will become much clearer as you read this chapter.

There have been some children who have not been ready to participate in a build partnership with a peer and have progressed to this via a number of sessions where the adult took the role of build partner and facilitator. For one particular case we have worked with, the child's skills and behaviour dictated the need for two adults in the session. One was his build partner and the other the facilitator. In this way it was possible to manipulate his partner's responses so that he gradually became more tolerant of errors and of waiting his turn. This then allowed him, eventually, to participate with a peer without meltdowns that had previously characterized his relationship with peers.

Role of the facilitator

Any intervention programme should have a clear theoretical foundation. It is essential for anyone delivering an intervention programme to know *what* they are targeting as well as *how* to carry out the intervention.

The model of language development proposed by Bloom and Lahey in 1978 (discussed in Chapter 1) can be used to consider the *what*.

Bloom and Lahey identify three connected language skills: 'content', 'form' and 'use', each of which needs to be well developed and coordinated for understanding, expression and successful communication.

LEGO® Therapy in its original form, first described by LeGoff (2004) and then by Owens *et al.* (2008), targets development of the *use* of language, as described by this model. Those who took part in the original therapy sessions were described as having 'adequate language' to participate in the activity. That is, they had developed adequate skills in the *content* and *form* of language but required intervention to develop its *use*.

Building Language Using LEGO® Bricks can be used with those who need help to develop any or all of these areas.

- Content:

    ○ Understanding and use of basic concepts of shape, size, position and colour.

- Form:
  - ○ Understanding and use of an increasing number of ICW.
  - ○ Combining words into phrases and sentences in grammatically correct ways.
- Use:
  - ○ Joint attention, turn taking, eye contact, communication repair and understanding of someone else's perspective (theory of mind) etc.

The role of the facilitator during a Building Language Using LEGO® Bricks session will vary depending upon the area of language development that is targeted. As this intervention can develop a wide range of skills it is vital that sessions are planned with clear aims in mind. Bloom and Lahey's model can be used to focus intervention on specific communication skills.

We do recognize that whilst it is useful to divide skills up to aid the facilitator in planning intervention sessions, it is likely that individuals participating in Building Language Using LEGO® Bricks will require intervention in more than one of these areas. The facilitator must, then, prioritize targets according to the need and the developmental stage of the children they are working with.

We have found, in our practice, that more than one target can be addressed at the same time. Again the number of targets set will depend upon the nature of the child's communication disorder, their build partner's skill level and the child's cognitive (learning) skills.

We will discuss the facilitator's role in relation to each of the skill areas of content, form and use. However, first we will discuss the use of prompts.

Prompting

Prompts are additional cues that we give the child to help them produce the response we are looking for. The facilitator's role is to provide the appropriate level of prompting to facilitate the desired skill and then gradually withdraw these prompts, so that the child is able to use the targeted skill independently. This process is called 'fading prompts'.

The use of systematically fading prompts is central to the success of Building Language Using LEGO® Bricks. Fading is a technique applied in behaviour modification where a prompt, initially needed to perform an action, is gradually withdrawn until the need for it fades. The overall aim is for the child to produce the action without the need for the prompt. In Building Language Using LEGO® Bricks the prompts are gradually faded from most intrusive to less intrusive and then withdrawn as the child becomes independent with the targeted skill.

Prompting in Building Language Using LEGO® Bricks differs slightly from the usual method of fading in that in the initial stages a number of prompts are combined, and then fading gradually withdraws these prompts, one by one, until the skill is established.

The hierarchy of prompts will differ depending upon whether you are targeting content, form or use. The hierarchy for fading prompts will be discussed in each of the sections below.

The prompts used will also depend upon the child's ability to divide their attention between visual and verbal stimuli. For some children with autism this is a difficult thing to do (single channelled attention). In this case the facilitator will have to explore which type of prompt is most useful in facilitating the desired response.

The prompts used include:

- *verbal* – a spoken word or prompt question

- *manual sign* or consistent gesture

- *visual image* – a picture or symbol.

We will discuss each of these prompt types in turn.

Verbal prompt

Spoken language is just strings of sounds that come to represent things in the world and their actions and relationships to each other. The relationship between a word and what it represents is arbitrary, for example, there is no reason why the sounds /c/ /a/ /t/, in spoken English, represents the furry animal that meows.

When a young child first starts to understand language they must listen to strings of connected speech sounds. They must pick out which sounds combine to make up words and then make the connection between the word and the 'thing' that it represents. If they consistently hear the sounds /c/ /a/ /t/ when their attention is drawn to the furry, meowing creature they will eventually associate these sounds with the creature and understanding of the word /cat/ will begin to develop. Knowledge of the word is then deepened and refined through a process called mapping (see Chapter 4) as the child encounters the word in a range of contexts.

Of all the prompting strategies, verbal or spoken prompts are the most transient. That is, they are only there for a fraction of a second and then rely on the child holding the word in their memory and processing it for meaning. For this reason, in early sessions, it can be useful to team a spoken prompt with a visual prompt that is less transient.

The level of verbal prompting will be dependent upon the child's language levels and the skills being targeted.

As a general rule, use simple sentence structures or single words where possible and always ensure that the child's attention is on the item you are naming.

Manual signing or consistent gesture

We have found signing to be an invaluable form of prompting for those with language impairment and also some on the autism spectrum. For some children with autism who are single channelled, it may be that using just the visual aids or spoken word suffices, as too many prompts may overload them. We have found, however, for most of the children we have worked with, that signing just the key words can really help with comprehension and use of language. Whilst this form of prompting is still transient, it tends to be more concrete than an arbitrary word. Take the Sign Supported English (SSE) sign for 'on' for example (the back of one hand placed on top of the other). This gesture makes the meaning of the word visually clear and thus supports understanding of a less concrete concept. The final hand posture can also be retained for longer than a spoken word, making it less transient.

Manual signing uses visual pathways to tap into language. Visual processing is often stronger than auditory processing in those with language impairment and those with autism. A sign alone can be used to prompt use of an emerging word. A signed question can prompt stages of the problem-solving process and signing can be used to support formulation of word order and grammatical structure.

There are a number of manual signing systems in existence. Some are dependent upon the country of origin, for example British Sign Language (BSL) as opposed to American Sign Language (ASL). Both of these are living languages and grow and change constantly as spoken languages do. They are also subject to dialectal changes in the way spoken language is. The grammatical structures used in both these languages differ from the spoken English.

There are also a number of signing systems that have developed specifically to support communication and language learning in those with language and learning difficulties. These include Makaton, Signalong and Paget-Gorman Signed Speech.

Makaton is a set of vocabulary based on what we most need to be able to communicate. There are signs and symbols for each of the words in this vocabulary set. The signs were originally drawn from BSL, however, some signs are now different due to the changing nature of BSL.

Signalong is again based on BSL. Signalong has also developed a wide range of signing resources to support the curriculum in schools.

Paget-Gorman Signed Speech is a concept-based system. Signs are grouped into categories, which helps to reinforce the natural organization of word learning, for example, all animal signs start with the same basic hand shape and slight alterations differentiate the different animals.

It does not matter which signing system is used to support language during Building Language Using LEGO® Bricks sessions. What is important is that the signs used are consistent – that the facilitator always uses the same sign for the same word. This ensures visual support for that transient spoken word.

As Building Language Using LEGO® Bricks is an intervention used to develop understanding and use of *spoken* language, it is vital that whatever signs are used follow the natural word order of that spoken language. It has been our practice to use SSE. This uses signs drawn from BSL but follows the word order of spoken English. It also provides grammatical markers for word endings like –ing, past tense –ed or plural –s, should these be needed.

There is a common concern amongst parents, that the use of signing will prevent a child from developing spoken language. This is definitely not the case. In fact, many studies have found the opposite effect. Signing facilitates the use of spoken language. It has been our experience that as soon as children are able to understand a spoken word or use speech, then signing is naturally dropped. This experience is supported by research findings. The following extract is taken from the *Resource Manual for Commissioning and Planning Services for SLCN* published by the Royal College of Speech and Language Therapists ('Learning Disability', Enderby *et al.* 2009 p.18).

> Millar (2006) undertook a systematic review to determine the effects of Augmentative and Alternative Communication (AAC) on speech production in individuals with developmental disabilities. Searches on electronic databases searching and key journals identified 23 studies. Six of the 23 studies were selected according to criteria specifying that inclusion of only those studies that established a comparison no treatment or alternative treatment group. Five studies investigated the effects of unaided AAC interventions, most specifically instruction in manual signs whilst the remaining study looked at an aided AAC system without speech output. 78% of the AAC interventions were highly structured and led by the speech and language therapist; the remainder were child-centred play activities. In total, the studies included 17 participants; four with autism and thirteen with mental retardation, Down's Syndrome or developmental delay. The mean number of sessions

was 42. In 89% of cases speech production increased with the mean number of words gained being 13. More importantly, no cases demonstrated a decrease in speech production post AAC intervention, indicating that AAC is not harmful to the speech production in individuals with developmental disabilities.

Readers are directed to a wealth of signing apps or websites available on the internet to learn how to sign key words. If signing is already used in the child's environment, for example at school, then this system should be used. As Building Language Using LEGO® Bricks is primarily aimed at facilitating language development, it is vital that the sign is always produced simultaneously with the spoken word.

Visual image

This can be the most powerful of all prompting systems, as visual images tap into visual processing, which, as discussed above, is usually a relative strength in the children we have worked with.

Visual images can be photographs, drawings or symbols. Photographs are conceptually the easiest visual image to understand and symbols (usually a line drawing) conceptually the most difficult. The child's visual perceptual skills and their cognitive development will determine which images they will find most supportive.

There are a number of recognized visual symbol systems that can be used to support understanding of spoken language. These include Makaton symbols, Widgit and Picture Communication System (PCS).

Any visual image will serve to support spoken language. You do not have to use one of these recognized systems. Most computers now have clip art available, which can be used to generate clear visual images for use in sessions. The most essential feature (as with any form of prompting) is that the same visual image is consistently used to represent each spoken word, concept or behaviour that you wish to reinforce.

Visual symbols can be used to prompt and reinforce understanding and use of words, concepts and social behaviour, like listening and waiting your turn. Symbols are very powerful tools to teach sequencing of ideas and language, for example we have used a series of symbols to prompt children to ensure they supply their build partner with all the information they need to understand a command. So instead of just saying 'blue', a sequence of symbols representing size, colour and then shape can prompt 'big, blue square'. Some symbols that we have produced ourselves and have found useful, during assessment and intervention, have been included in the appendices of this book. We hope that you will find it useful to photocopy these and use them to support the needs of the children you are working with.

Facilitating use of language

The role of the facilitator in using Building Language Using LEGO® Bricks to develop socially appropriate use of language is similar to that described in the original research (LeGoff, 2004). Therapy should move along a smooth continuum from adult-directed communication to peer mediation. As with all areas of this intervention, the facilitator will have to intervene more frequently during the initial sessions but will gradually 'step back' and allow the participants to work out social solutions more independently as the intervention progresses.

Children are able to communicate long before they develop the form and content of their language. They are born with a repertoire of skills that help them to have their basic needs met, like crying and wriggling. They then quickly develop use of eye contact and gesture to communicate their needs. Initially the children are unaware of the communicative effect of these skills, however, through the consistent response of their caregiver they are quickly shaped into communicative routines.

Through ongoing interaction with people around them children learn 'communicative competence', that is, how to use language appropriately and strategically in social situations. To acquire social competence, children need to learn to use language for a wide variety of functions. These include: asking questions, making requests, agreeing, disagreeing, refusing, apologizing, telling stories, reporting events, praising others and engaging people in conversation. Children must learn how to initiate, maintain and terminate conversations in 'polite' ways. They must stay on the same topic as their communication partner and learn how to take turns appropriately.

One of the most important skills children must learn is to be sensitive to 'who' they are speaking to and to the situation they are communicating in. Consider the different ways a child would speak to a teacher or to a friend; also the way a child would speak in the playground or in the cinema. Children develop more sophisticated 'use of language' throughout childhood and into adulthood.

Social problem solving is a vital skill for successful social integration in most situations and is vital to the development of social competence.

If you were to ask me my name and you then misheard my answer and called me by a different name, the way that I corrected you would determine how our relationship progressed. Consider:

> 'No stupid! I didn't say that!'

Or:

> 'Sorry I think you misheard me, my name is actually…'

The problem-solving process used in this situation is universal to all settings.

1. Identify a problem.

2. Ascertain the nature of the problem.

3. Formulate a socially appropriate solution.

4. Test out the solution.

5. Shape your response based on the listener's reaction.

The main feature of the facilitator's role when developing use of language is to prompt participants through this problem-solving process.

- Help participants identify when there is a problem: 'Did John do what you asked?'

- Prompt them to identify the nature of the problem: 'Why not?' 'What went wrong?'

- Prompt them to form solutions: 'How could we help him listen?'

- Help them to try the solution: 'Yes, say his name and wait until he looks at you.'

- Reinforce good use of solutions with the use of a token: 'Well done, you called his name first.'

- Remind participants of successful strategies used in the past so that they can be generalized to other situations: 'What helped him listen last time?'

Consistent use of this step-by-step prompting can result in the child internalizing this problem-solving process so that it can be applied to other social situations. It is vital that participants are aided in generating their own solutions and can try these out in the safety of the session to see if they are effective.

The facilitator must, then, be sensitive to when prompting is needed and when to withdraw the prompt and wait for a solution to be reached independently.

For some children, visual representations of the steps of this problem-solving process, in the form of symbols or written words, can be used as a bridge between facilitator prompting and independent social problem-solving. Versions that we have used are provided in Appendix 9.

Verbal prompting is used throughout sessions to help identify the initial stage of the problem-solving process. In the initial stages questions are used to focus participants' attention on the problem-solving process:

- 'Is that right?'

- 'What is wrong?'

- 'What can you do to help him?'

- 'What could you say?'

- 'What does he need to do?'

Tokens are a very powerful tool that helps the facilitator draw attention to the use of skills that are being targeted. Tokens can be awarded for any behaviour that is moving towards the desired outcome. So, for example, any move to the first step of problem solving (identification of a problem) can be instantly pointed out and reinforced by awarding a token. Tokens can then be used, combined with verbal and visual prompting, to gradually shape skills towards a more complete solution.

We have found the following sequence of fading cues useful in the development of 'use'.

1. Full prompting of the targeted skill, verbal, sign and symbols.

2. Token reinforcement of the facilitated skill.

3. Gradually reduce prompting to sign and symbol.

4. Token reinforcement of the facilitated skill.

5. Reduce prompting to sign only.

6. Token reinforcement of the facilitated skill.

7. Prompt by a questioning look or a verbal (or signed) question 'What?' *What should you do now?*

8. Token reinforcement of the facilitated skill.

9. As the skill becomes established gradually fade the use of tokens so that you only token the skill intermittently.

10. Once the skill is well established omit tokens and move on to another skill, as the motivation to complete the action will be intrinsic.

Anything can be used as a token reward during Building Language Using LEGO® Bricks sessions. We have used small paper tokens, which are included in Appendix 11 for your use. We suggest that these are laminated and used in all sessions.

We have given up to 50 tokens in a session, so make sure you have plenty available. The tokens have not led to a further reward. We count tokens at the end of the session and then place them back in a container for use next time. Some children like to keep a record of the number of tokens they have collected.

Facilitating content of language

The content of a language, according to Bloom and Lahey's model is the meaning that is expressed through words (semantics). There are many categories of meaning that are expressed as we communicate with others (some of these are objects, actions, relations between things).

A child usually utters their first meaningful word around their first birthday; however, there is a wide variety in developmental norms at this stage, ranging from about 8 months to 16 months. Children have been exposed to a lot of language by this stage and usually have a receptive vocabulary (words they understand) of about 50 words (Bates *et al.*, 1994). As children learn more words they move from the concrete names of things and people to complex, abstract and relational concepts such as words for actions, emotions and colours. Children make connections between the words they learn, building a complex network of interrelated words and concepts. This lexical development carries on into adulthood as we continue to add new words (e.g. selfie) (see Chapter 4).

Building Language Using LEGO® Bricks is a powerful intervention to develop content by facilitating a growing understanding of the concepts needed to describe the bricks, their location and the actions needed to achieve the build.

Chapter 5 describes test procedures to establish a baseline of skills in relation to concept development. This can then be used to develop a progression for teaching these concepts.

The facilitator's role in relation to developing content is to provide the child with sufficient prompts and supports to enable them to understand the concepts being expressed through their build partner's language. They must then gradually fade these prompts so that the child can understand the concept from the spoken word alone. The sequence for fading prompts is given below. This can be used to teach understanding of a word (that represents a concept) or use of a spoken concept word.

1. Full prompting of the targeted skill, verbal, sign and symbols.

2. Token reinforcement of understanding or use of the word.

3. Gradually reduce prompting to sign and spoken word.

4. Token reinforcement of understanding or use of the word.

5. Reduce prompting to spoken word only.

6. Token reinforcement of understanding or use of the word.

7. As the skill becomes established gradually fade the use of tokens so that you only token the skill intermittently.

8. Once the skill is well established omit tokens and move on to another word.

Generally speaking, understanding of a word develops before it is used, so it makes sense to teach a child to understand a given concept word before you expect them to use it to give directions to their partner. With this in mind, you may find that in order to stimulate use of a word that the child has just learned to understand, you may need to revert to a higher level of prompting. These prompts can then be faded (as above) as the word becomes established in the child's repertoire.

Facilitating form of language

The form of a language is how it is constructed: the rules that govern how speech sounds combine to form words (phonology) and how words combine to form sentences, that is word order and grammatical structure (syntax). It also includes how we use morphemes, the smallest units of meaning. These include suffixes and prefixes that add meaning, like plural –s or past tense –ed (morphology).

Children learn early on that rule-based combinations of words can convey more meaning than the words alone, for example, Golinkoff *et al.* (1996) found that children as young as 17 months could understand the difference between 'Cookie Monster is tickling Big Bird' and 'Big Bird is tickling Cookie Monster'.

Building Language Using LEGO® Bricks can address some of the features of form by gradually increasing the number of ICW that can be understood and used. Again, verbal and visual prompts are used to move the child from single word responses to connected speech. Correct word order and grammatical features can be prompted and rehearsed through the repetitive format of a build activity.

Sequences of symbols can be used to prompt the correct order of concepts. So when directing a build partner to select the correct brick we would usually say, 'get the big, blue square' as opposed to 'get the square, big, blue'. This sequence can be prompted by the use of a symbol strip depicting /size/colour/shape/ (see Appendix 7).

Building Language Using LEGO® Bricks can be used as a medium to gradually increase the number of ICW that the child is able to hold in their auditory memory in order to process a spoken direction. It is the facilitator's role to manipulate the environment so that the instruction given by the build partner is at the correct ICW level for each child. This manipulation can take two forms.

- Provide sign or visual image prompts for some of the words, thus reducing the pressure on auditory memory.

- Offer a reduced selection of bricks to choose from, which negates the need to understand some of the concepts.

So, if the instruction was, 'get the big, blue square', then depending on context, each of the words 'big', 'blue' and 'square' could be an ICW (3 ICW level).

To reduce this to a 2 ICW level the facilitator could do the following.

- Point to the symbol for /big/ as the instruction is given, leaving just 'blue' and 'square' to be held in auditory memory. To do this it is often necessary to ask the build partner to repeat the direction as you point to the symbol.

- Offer only big bricks, thus negating the need to process the concept of size. It is vital that you ensure there are alternatives for the other concepts of 'blue' and 'square' to ensure this remains a 2 ICW level. Choices could be: a big, blue square; a big, red square; a big, blue rectangle; a big, red rectangle. You can change the alternatives you offer to match your targets. So, if you were working on the concept of size you could offer big and little bricks but only offer a single colour (blue) or a single shape (rectangle).

By gradually manipulating the ICW level, children can be pushed towards a higher level of challenge. We have found that the motivation of achieving the build has resulted in rapid changes in this area.

The instructions given during a build tend to be repetitive ('get the big, red rectangle', 'put it on the flat, white square). This lends itself to the development of correct grammatical structure through the process of modelling and prompting. We have found that children who usually omit function words like 'the', 'is', 'a', begin to use these when giving instructions after a few sessions of modelling. Signing these small words can be very useful in the initial stages to prompt their use. Other evidence-based approaches to developing grammatical structure can be used to prompt correct structures when giving instructions, for example Shape Coding (Ebbels, 2007) could be used to provide a visual template for these repetitive sentence structures.

Choosing a build model

The choice of model is one of the most important factors influencing the success of this intervention. Our experience has indicated that the following criteria should be considered.

- Attention control: The child's attention span will dictate the amount of time they can focus on the activity. This influences the number of stages in each build. Moving through a series of gradually lengthening builds can increase attention span. The patience (or tolerance for waiting for a response) of the build partner will also influence the length of the build. Again, as patience increases, the number of steps in the build can be gradually increased.

- Fine motor control: The child's ability to manipulate the bricks physically will dictate the size of the bricks used. If the child presents with difficulties in this area the build is likely to take longer and thus fewer steps may be required initially to ensure a build is completed.

- Tolerating an incomplete build: Most children (especially those on the autism spectrum) find it difficult to leave a build incomplete. Many times, in the school environment and outside, we are required to stop activities before they are complete. For children on the autism spectrum this can cause high levels of anxiety. We have successfully worked on increasing tolerance through gradually moving from builds that can be completed in one session to those that will take several sessions to complete. In order to do this the build has to be carefully selected so we can determine how many sessions it will take. We can then 'warn' the children of this and set up strategies to help them cope.

The following strategies have proved successful.

- Warn the children how many sessions the build will take. Very gradually build this, starting with one, then two etc.

- Take a photograph of the part built model and reassure the child that it will remain unchanged until the next session. The child can be given the photograph to keep if this helps.

- Place the incomplete model in a cupboard (this can be locked if needed) and reassure the child that no one will touch the model before the next session. Our experience has been that, in the early stages, the children may ask to see the model to reassure themselves it is unchanged. We always honour this request. Trust usually builds quickly and these strategies can be gradually faded out.

- Targets: The targets selected for each child will influence the build. Targets to increase the use of communication repair strategies dictate the need for communication to break down. Thus a model that is slightly above the level that the children can achieve independently will mean that incidents of communication breakdown will occur, thus creating opportunities for prompting repair strategies.

Targeted language concepts will dictate how the build proceeds, particularly the sequencing of instructions. For example, let's say we were building a house. If targeting the concept 'in front of', we would start the build at the back of the construction so that each subsequent brick in a wall had to be placed 'in front of' the last brick. In this way you can give many exposures to the targeted concept. If the target was 'behind', then the reverse would be needed. Start the wall at the front of the construction and work backwards so that the word 'behind' is used as much as possible. The same model can be used for many concepts. Just the sequence of instructions is changed. This can be achieved by first building the model in the sequence you require and then photographing and numbering each stage of the build. We have included a checklist in Appendix 2 so you can note which concepts etc. are challenged by which instruction set. This makes planning easier in the long term. We recognize that following the criteria above can be time consuming and difficult when your time is pressured. Rest assured that any model will offer opportunities to target many language skills. All models address non-verbal communication and use of language skills. The criteria above are useful in ensuring your quickest route to reaching targets.

Every model works on developing joint attention throughout the activity. If this is the primary target then any build that the children are motivated to do will help achieve this.

Chapter 7

Guidelines for Setting Up and Running Building Language Using LEGO® Bricks Sessions

Building Language Using LEGO® Bricks in school

Below are helpful guidelines on how to run sessions. These are what worked for us, but are not prescriptive. You may want to run your groups differently. Please go with whatever works for you and your client group and do not feel bound to follow our format.

Before starting sessions, you will need suitable builds and instruction sets. We have found that for some children the instructions that come in ready-made sets can be a little confusing. They are often visually complex and may include several steps in one stage. We have found it useful either to create our own models or use bought model sets but make new instructions. We have done this by building the model and photographing each new brick addition. These steps are numbered and form the instructions.

If the child can work from the LEGO® instructions booklet a handy tip is to cover all but the current step with sticky notes. This reduces visual clutter.

- Find a quiet room with minimal distractions that is available at the same time each week. If this is a room that is sometimes used for other activities, e.g. speech and language or occupational therapy, it may be helpful to put a sign up so that the activity is clear.

- We recommend a minimum of 40 minutes per session, as this gives time for each child to experience each role for 15 minutes plus some extra time for greetings, rules, problem solving, model play etc.

- Decide on the best way to time exchanging of roles. We would recommend something tangible like a sand timer or a clock. Alternatively, you could agree a set number of turns for each child in a given role.

- We have found videoing the sessions invaluable. It is so easy to miss subtle changes in both verbal and non-verbal communication while in the sessions, as we are so involved in facilitation. We have used the videos to complete the assessment forms and to mark progress. We always ask the children's permission and give them the opportunity to watch some of the footage either at the end of the session or at a later date. Parental permission for videoing is always sought.

All sessions follow a predictable format so that those children who rely on structure quickly relax into the session. This format is as follows.

1. Practise greeting group members.

2. Introduce activity.

3. Introduce Building Language Using LEGO® Bricks rules.

4. Practise language needed (naming bricks, positional language etc.).

5. Introduce tokens.

6. Build model.

7. Tidy up and self-evaluation sheet.

8. Goodbyes.

First session

- Please refer to Chapter 6 for details of how to assist during the sessions. Ensure you are familiar with the sequence for fading prompts depending upon the skills you are targeting.

- Start by telling the children what Building Language Using LEGO® Bricks is. Keep the explanation as simple as possible. Use signing and visual prompts where appropriate. The following is an example of the explanation:

  > We are going to build models together. You have to listen to each other and talk to each other to build a LEGO® model. You will take it in turns to give the instructions and to do the building. I am going to help you to do this and we are going to have lots of fun. You will get tokens every time that you do something well and we will count them up at the end to see how many you have.

For some children we have reduced this explanation to very short statements and relied on experiential learning.

- Explain each of the roles and show the badges:

  > 'The engineer has the instructions and tells the builder what bricks are needed to build a model.' (The builder can't see the instructions.)
  > 'The builder listens to the engineer and uses the bricks to build a model.'
  > 'Every session, you will take it in turns to be the engineer and the builder.'

- Introduce the rules. Sometimes the rules are generic and other times it may be helpful to write them with a particular behaviour in mind, e.g. hitting or chair throwing.

- For the first session we recommend choosing a very basic model containing no more than six steps. We always use a model using DUPLO® bricks that we have built and photographed ourselves. This model contains squares and rectangles and only primary colours. Place the bricks the correct way up and group them according to their colours. The first session needs to be simple and achievable, especially when working with children whose self-esteem may be low and anxiety high.

- Practise the language needed for each build. Decide on terms that could be ambiguous, e.g. what would you call the raised dots that join the bricks together? If the children use a specific term follow their lead.

- Role assignment. We have found that most of the children want to be the builder and this is where early negotiation skills (or lack of) are tested. For the first few sessions, it may be easier to assign the roles for the children, as this is a skill that has to be modelled and practised. Interestingly, we have noticed that it does not take long for the children to realize that if they are the builder last, they might get to put the wheels on a model, which rates highly in satisfaction levels when building a model.

- Model the language for the engineer and use the visual prompt strip to demonstrate the order, e.g.: 'You need…' *or* 'Find…'

    Ask the engineer to repeat, and give a token to the engineer for 'good asking' and a token to the builder for 'good listening' when they have found the correct piece.

    Model the language again: 'Well done. Put it on the table. Find the green square.'

    Again, once the engineer has requested and the builder has found the correct piece, give a token to each.

    'Yes. Put the green square on the blue square.'

    Continue using simple language and modelling correct responses. If you are using a six-brick build, remind the children that they will be swapping roles after three photos/ instructions.

- Sometimes the children themselves want to move chairs so that it is easier for them to switch roles or they may be fine with just swapping their badges over. Continue again with modelling the language and responses, whilst awarding tokens throughout.

- The children tend to ask the adult for confirmation that they are correct. If this is the case, direct them to ask their build partner either verbally, e.g. 'ask John' or by pointing.

- When the build is finished, congratulate the children on working together to build a first model. Take a photo of it, if you can, as it will be a great baseline record for measuring what they will, it is hoped, go on to achieve in the following few sessions. The children often like to show the photographs to other adults and peers. They can also be sent home.

- Ask the children to fill in their evaluation sheet (Appendix 12) by ticking one of the boxes. If they are able to, they can write something about their first session or you can scribe for them.

- Ask/help the children to count up their tokens (Appendix 11). They can write the amount on their evaluation sheet if they want to keep a record.

- Tell them that the session has finished and ask the children to help tidy the bricks away.

- Prompt goodbyes to their build partner and yourself.

Subsequent sessions

- Continue with the same format so that consistency runs throughout each session: greetings, rules,* role allocation etc. The aim is for the children to be able to facilitate this independently without the need for reminders. Practising this every session using visual/verbal/signing prompts and tokens will make it start to flow more naturally.

*After a few sessions, it may not be necessary to repeat the rules if they are generic and not specific to a behaviour. Instead, the rules can be pinned up and referred to only if needed.

- Until the children's confidence grows, use simple models that can be finished within a session. This may continue over a few weeks while the relationship builds between the children. As mentioned previously, it can be a difficult thing to leave a model unfinished and this has got to be timed correctly. You should find that the need for modelling language reduces as the children's skills and confidence grow.

- Progress the children onto more 'difficult' builds as their skills improve. As the sessions will be very much 'needs led', the builds you choose will depend upon a number of factors. These will include: language skills and targets, fine motor and bilateral integration skills, cognitive development and attention control (see 'Choosing a build model' in Chapter 6). Don't be tempted to progress to more difficult builds too quickly. Go at the child's rate of progress. It may be that the children only ever build models using DUPLO® bricks. Your skills as a model builder and photographer will be put to good use!

- Review targets with the children and help them to set their own targets if possible, e.g. 'I will recognize a rectangle from a group of shapes four out of five times,' or 'I will use a full sentence when giving my partner instructions.'

- After each session, take a photograph of the finished model so that there is a record of their achievements. It can be difficult for some children to destroy their build after a session, although for some this is the best bit. Taking a photograph of the model can make this easier to accept.

- Please see Chapter 6 for detailed guidance on the facilitator's role, as this will talk you through how to reduce your input and increase the children's language and communication skills.

Building Language Using LEGO® Bricks at home

We are often asked by parents and carers if Building Language Using LEGO® Bricks is something that they can do with their children at home. So often play, especially for a child with autism, is a solitary activity and parents and carers can feel isolated from their children. One of the concerns usually raised is how to make the transition from what the child usually does (engage in solitary construction tasks) with LEGO® bricks to the paired cooperative format of Building Language Using LEGO® Bricks, without eliciting a meltdown.

One of the suggestions that appears to have been successful is to 'dress up' Building Language Using LEGO® Bricks as a new game. See below for details.

1. Choose a model that your child is not familiar with.

2. Label up a box with whatever you would like to call the 'game', e.g. 'Building Fun', 'Dad and *Charlie's* Building Game'.

3. Keep the model and all of the visual prompts and visual aids in the box along with the rules of the game and tokens.

4. You are more than likely going to have some LEGO® bricks in the house already so keep the 'game' separate from it so that your child knows that there is a difference.

5. Our belief is that it will be more difficult to build a model over a series of weeks at home, especially if your child has autism. Rules that they may accept at school may be too difficult to adhere to at home, where free-play is always allowed. If this is the case, try to find or create models that can be finished in one sitting. Your child is more likely to want to repeat this activity with you if they are not frustrated or angry at the end of the session. As well as the benefits of improving language and communication, your main aim at home is probably to connect with your child on their level and play jointly with them.

Most parents have facilitated Building Language Using LEGO® Bricks sessions between siblings, however it could just as easily be an activity that could be used during play dates to help foster the building of relationships between peers.

In some instances, the parent has been both facilitator and build partner. This is sometimes an initial step that is needed in order to move the child to a stage where they can succeed with their sibling or another child.

See above for step-by-step instructions of how to carry out the initial session.

Chapter 8

Measuring Outcomes

The Bercow Report (2008, p.12) noted that: 'A continual cycle of self evaluation is required in order to improve outcomes.'

It is vital, then, that when working with children or adults we can show that any intervention we use is doing what we were hoping it would do. In the case of Building Language Using LEGO® Bricks, we need to show that it is helping to develop the language and communication skills of those we are working with.

Target-based outcomes

There are many 'outcome measures' used within health and education that can be applied to this approach, for example, Goal Attainment Scale (GAS) or East Kent Outcome System (EKOS) (Johnson and Elias, 2010). Readers must choose whichever system is most appropriate for their particular setting. What is common to most is that we must first identify exactly what we expect the child to achieve by setting a SMART target. SMART stands for the following.

- **S**pecific – target a specific area for improvement, e.g. X will learn to understand the concept 'behind' in relation to their own perspective.

- **M**easured – success should be quantified or at least there should be an indicator of progress, e.g. X will consistently be able to place a brick behind another brick when given a simple 1 ICW instruction by their build partner in nine out of ten trials.

- **A**ppropriate or **A**ttainable – making sure that target is within the child's potential given the level and frequency of input to achieve it.

- **R**elevant – if a child is unable to turn take and does not yet understand the concept 'beside', it is likely that turn taking would be a more relevant goal as it is fundamental to many communication situations. However, if the child was failing to understand a curriculum topic in class because of their lack of understanding of the concept 'beside' this then may take priority, as it would be more relevant to that child's needs at that point in time.

- **T**imed – specific as to when the target will be achieved, e.g. X will place a brick behind another in response to their build partner's 1 ICW instruction, by the end of six Building Language Using LEGO® Bricks sessions.

In order to set a SMART target, we must first establish what the child is able to do (a baseline of skills). We can then look at the next step we would like them to develop.

To aid with establishing a baseline, we have provided a description of informal test procedures for many of the language skills that are targeted through the use of this intervention (see Chapter 5). These should be coupled with observation of the child's performance within sessions to ensure you keep an ongoing assessment of their level of skill.

The assessment checklists provided in the appendices can be used to record test results or observations. We have included columns for understanding (comprehension) of a given word or skill (comp) and use (expression) of that word or skill (expr). We have found it useful to complete this checklist prior to a block of Building Language Using LEGO® Bricks sessions and then once this block has been completed.

Some children may progress more slowly due to the severity of their language or cognitive deficits. In this case, progress towards the target may be measured by a reduction in prompt dependency. In order to make the checklist more sensitive to change, an agreed system of abbreviations could be used to record the level of prompting needed to elicit the targeted skill. We would suggest the following:

- M = skill mastered
- E = skill emerging
- N = not yet aware.

E could be further qualified by noting which prompts are needed to elicit the target, using the following abbreviations:

- Sp = spoken word
- S = sign
- V = visual (symbol or picture).

Targets can then be set to reflect this progression, for example X will understand the word 'behind' in a 1 ICW instruction given the spoken word and sign. The next target will then be spoken word alone.

Completion of the checklists prior to the sessions allows us to establish a baseline of skills and thus set child-specific targets for intervention. We can then manipulate which builds we offer the child and how the facilitator will work in each session according to these targets (see Chapter 6 for details).

Completion of the checklist after a block of sessions allows us to evaluate if the child has achieved their targets and thus draw conclusions about how effective the intervention has been.

Use of the checklist and test procedures coupled with post-intervention retesting can provide valuable data about the efficacy of the intervention and the child's rate of progress. This can then be used to inform further interventions.

This information when used in conjunction with either GAS, EKOS or similar target-based systems can generate data, which can be shared with commissioners of services.

Satisfaction-based outcomes

As well as target-centred outcomes, we also measure satisfaction or enjoyment ratings using a simple questionnaire. This has been included for your use in Appendix 12. The children complete this at the end of each session. We have tended to offer this questionnaire as part of the routine of the session, however, if a child expresses a wish not to complete it we, of course, respect this but still offer it at the end of each subsequent session.

Chapter 9

Examples of Cases

Please note that we are not presenting actual case studies in this chapter. Instead we believe that it would be more useful to provide examples of how to use Building Language Using LEGO® Bricks with children with a wide range of disabilities. Between us, we have over 30 years of experience of working with children and young adults with complex needs. We believe that we can use our knowledge to provide a guide of how best to introduce Building Language Using LEGO® Bricks as a successful intervention.

Some of the characteristics of the fictional case studies that we will present will reflect those of children with whom we have worked. They are, however, an amalgamation of many children, so that we can provide case studies that will be the most useful. The names that we use in the case studies are purely fictional.

These cases will take you through from assessment and target setting to model building and progression.

John
Background information
Chronological age: 11

Diagnosis: John is described as having Speech, Language and Communication Needs (SLCN) within the context of learning difficulties, however his Education Health Care Plan (EHCP) states that his SLCN are his primary need.

John has clear speech and can speak in short phrases, although these are immature for his age. His understanding of language is limited for his chronological age.

John is described as having limited attention control and is slow to learn new words.

John does not present with any impairment of fine motor control. He would be able to manipulate smaller LEGO® bricks.

John is sociable and likes to play with others but, due to his difficulties understanding and using language, he tends to play with those much younger than himself.

Assessment

The informal assessment activities described in Chapter 5 were carried out.

John was also observed at break time, at school and in the classroom.

Information from these sources was used to complete the assessment checklists in Appendix 1. Completed checklists are below.

Note that not all concepts were tested (these are left blank). Once a significant area of deficit was identified, it was decided that these skills should be targeted. Further assessment may be carried out at a later date.

Often, observation of skills during sessions can give a clear idea of concept knowledge, without having to specifically test each concept individually.

Concept development

Colour	Pre intervention		Post intervention	
	comp	expr	comp	expr
Red	M	M		
Green	M	M		
Blue	M	M		
Yellow	M	M		
Black	M	M		
White	M	M		
Orange	M	M		
Brown	M	M		
Pink	M	M		
Purple	M	M		
Grey	M	M		
Light	N	N		
Dark	N	N		

Shape	Pre intervention		Post intervention	
	comp	expr	comp	expr
Square	M	M		
Rectangle	M	M		
Triangle	M	M		
Circle	M	M		
Slope	N	N		
Curve	N	N		
Semi circle	N	N		

Size	Pre intervention		Post intervention	
	comp	expr	comp	expr
Big	M	M		
Little	M	M		
Large	N	N		
Small	M	M		
Long	M	M		
Short (length)	M	M		
Thin				
Fat				
Flat	N	N		
Tall	N	N		
Short (height)	N	N		
Tiny	M	M		
Medium				

Sequences	Pre intervention		Post intervention	
	comp	expr	comp	expr
Before	N	N		
After	N	N		
Start	M	M		
Finish	M	M		
Change	N	N		
First				
Next				
Last				

Position	Pre intervention		Post intervention	
	comp	expr	comp	expr
On	M	M		
Under	M	M		
Between	N	N		
In	M	M		
Next to	M	M		
Beside				
In front of	N	N		
Behind	N	N		
End				
Middle				
Corner				
Edge				
Left				
Right				
Centre				
Opposite				
Other side				
Front	M	M	For objects with a clear front and back	
Back	M	M		
Move				
Turn				

Other

	Pre intervention		Post intervention	
	comp	expr	comp	expr
Numbers 1–5	M	M		
Numbers 5–10	M	M		
Numbers 10–20	M	M		
Numbers 20 plus				
Smooth				
Bumpy/rough				
Shiny				
Transparent/clear				
More				
Less				
Same				
Different				
Another				

Information-carrying words

	Pre intervention		Post intervention	
	comp	expr	comp	expr
1 ICW	M	M		
2 ICW	M	M		
3 ICW	N	N		
4 ICW				
5 ICW				

Question words

	Pre intervention		Post intervention	
	comp	expr	comp	expr
What?	M	M		
Where?	M	M		
Which?	M	N		
How?				
How many?				

Repair strategies

	Pre intervention		Post intervention	
	comp	expr	comp	expr
Gain/regain attention	M	M		
Request repetition	M	N		
Ask question	M	M		
Seek confirmation	N	N		
Ask for help from adult		M		
Ask for help from peer	N	N		

Non-verbal communication skills

	Pre intervention		Post intervention	
	comp	expr	comp	expr
Appropriate eye contact	M	M		
Joint attention	M	M		
Patience	M	M		
Turn taking	M	M		
Problem solving	N	N		

Summary of assessment results

John understands and uses some basic concept words needed for Building Language Using LEGO® Bricks. He knows most of his colours but does not yet understand the concept of light and dark in relation to colour shade.

He also knows and can name most of his basic shapes but does not know what a curve or a slope is.

He understands and uses some basic size concepts but does not yet understand the terms large, tall, short (height) and flat (opposite of a wide or fat brick).

John also understands some positional language but needs to develop his understanding of the words between, in front of and behind.

He understands and can name numbers up to 20.

John can only understand instructions requiring him to hold up to two ICW in his memory for processing. He cannot hold three ICW.

John understands and uses some question words.

John shows good use of most non-verbal communication skills but struggles with problem solving. However, his repair strategies, when communication breaks down, are limited.

Target setting
TARGETS

- John will understand the word 'large' in a 1 ICW instruction from his build partner (with no prompts) in a session, by the end of Session 4 with 95 per cent accuracy.

- John will understand the concept 'in front of' in a 1 ICW instruction from his build partner (with no prompts) in a session, by the end of Session 8, with 95 per cent accuracy.

- John will understand a 3 ICW instruction from his build partner (with no prompts) in a session, by the end of Session 8, with 95 per cent accuracy.

The principles of SMART targets should be followed (see Chapter 8). These helped us to choose where to start with target setting. The process is detailed below.

The targets above are all written to be: **S**pecific, **M**easured and **T**ime bound.

A for Attainable: As John already knows the word 'big' it was decided that 'large' would be a good word to select. Big can be used as a synonym to large to explain its meaning. We felt this meant that John would be able to achieve this target within a couple of sessions. This rapid progress is very motivating for a child and will ensure his future engagement in the sessions.

John understands the concepts of 'front' and 'back' in relation to himself and objects with a clear front and back. This knowledge can be used as a stepping stone to teaching the concepts of 'in front of' and 'behind'. As building bricks do not have a clear front and back, John will need to be taught how to understand this concept in relation to his own perspective. We have found it useful to teach that when he can see the whole face of the brick that is 'in front' and when the brick is partially or totally eclipsed that is 'behind'. The symbols included in Appendix 6 also support this view.

As John is able to understand 2 ICW instructions, moving him to 3 ICW instructions with fading prompts should be attainable.

R is for Relevant: Large is a word often used within the curriculum so is a relevant target to increase access to many lessons.

'In front of' is used in many areas of the curriculum. John is currently covering dance in his PE lessons and this preposition is used in this lesson.

Understanding of 3 ICW will greatly improve his comprehension in all settings so is very relevant.

Choosing a build partner

The build partner would need to have language skills that allow them to use the words 'large' and 'in front of' and to give 3 ICW instructions. They would therefore have language skills at a higher level than John.

John is likely to require extended processing time to respond to instructions. The build partner would either need to have developed tolerance of this or have this set as a target.

The build partner chosen for John is James, see below for details.

James

Background information

Chronological age: 12

Diagnosis: James was diagnosed with autism at the age of three years. He speaks in grammatically correct sentences and is able to use language at a higher level than John. James likes to talk about his special interests and can become frustrated easily. When James is anxious or frustrated he relies on adult intervention to stay calm. James doesn't recognize other people's needs and so is not tolerant when interacting with peers.

Assessment

The informal assessment activities described in Chapter 5 were carried out.

James was also observed at break time, at school and in the classroom.

Information from these sources was used to complete the assessment checklists in Appendix 1. Completed checklists follow.

As with John, not all concepts were tested (these were left blank). When a significant area of deficit was detected it was decided to target these skills.

Concept development

Colour	Pre intervention		Post intervention	
	comp	expr	comp	expr
Red	M	M		
Green	M	M		
Blue	M	M		
Yellow	M	M		
Black	M	M		
White	M	M		
Orange	M	M		
Brown	M	M		
Pink	M	M		
Purple	M	M		
Grey	M	M		
Light	M	M		
Dark	M	M		

Shape	Pre intervention		Post intervention	
	comp	expr	comp	expr
Square	M	M		
Rectangle	M	M		
Triangle	M	M		
Circle	M	M		
Slope	M	M		
Curve	M	M		
Semi circle	M	M		

Size	Pre intervention		Post intervention	
	comp	expr	comp	expr
Big	M	M		
Little	M	M		
Large	M	M		
Small	M	M		
Long	M	M		
Short (length)	M	M		
Thin	M	M		
Fat				
Flat	M	M		
Tall	M	M		
Short (height)	M	M		
Tiny	M	M		
Medium	M	M		

Sequences	Pre intervention		Post intervention	
	comp	expr	comp	expr
Before	E	N		
After	E	N		
Start	M	M		
Finish	M	M		
Change	M	M		
First	M	M		
Next	M	M		
Last	M	M		

Position	Pre intervention		Post intervention	
	comp	expr	comp	expr
On	M	M		
Under	M	M		
Between	M	M		
In	M	M		
Next to	M	M		
Beside	E	N		
In front of	M	M		
Behind	M	M		
End	E	E	Understand on objects with a definite start and end. Knows end of activity. Not sure with items with no obvious start and end (e.g. a line or a bridge).	
Middle	M	M		
Corner	M	M		
Edge	E	E		
Left	M	M	In relation to self but not others or objects from another person's perspective.	
Right	M	M		
Centre	N	N		
Opposite	E	E		
Other side	E	E		
Front	M	M		
Back	M	M		
Move	M	M		
Turn				

Other

	Pre intervention		Post intervention	
	comp	expr	comp	expr
Numbers 1–5	M	M		
Numbers 5–10	M	M		
Numbers 10–20	M	M		
Numbers 20 plus	M	M		
Smooth	M	M		
Bumpy/rough	M	M		
Shiny	M	M		
Transparent/clear	M	M	Understands/ uses clear but not transparent.	
More	M	M		
Less	M	M		
Same	M	M		
Different	M	M		
Another	M	M		

Information-carrying words

	Pre intervention		Post intervention	
	comp	expr	comp	expr
1 ICW	M	M		
2 ICW	M	M		
3 ICW	M	M		
4 ICW	E	E		
5 ICW				

Question words

	Pre intervention		Post intervention	
	comp	expr	comp	expr
What?	M	M		
Where?	M	M		
Which?	M	M		
How?	M	M		
How many?	M	M		

Repair strategies

	Pre intervention		Post intervention	
	comp	expr	comp	expr
Gain/regain attention	M	E		
Request repetition	M	N		
Ask question	M	M		
Seek confirmation	M	N		
Ask for help from adult	M	M		
Ask for help from peer	E	N		

Non-verbal communication skills

	Pre intervention		Post intervention	
	comp	expr	comp	expr
Appropriate eye contact	M	M	Mastered to a level that is comfortable for James and acceptable for communication.	
Joint attention	E	E		
Patience	N	N		
Turn taking	E	E		
Social problem solving	N	N		

Summary of assessment results

James understands and uses most of the concepts needed for sessions. His understanding of the concepts before, after, beside, opposite, other side and edge are emerging.

James's greatest area of need is with the 'use' of language (Bloom and Lahey model). He needs to develop his non-verbal communication skills in the following areas:

- joint attention
- patience
- turn taking
- social problem solving.

He also needs to develop his repair strategies:

- gain attention in socially appropriate ways
- request repetition
- seek confirmation
- ask a peer for help.

Target setting
TARGETS

- James will understand the word 'beside' in a 1 ICW instruction from his build partner (with no prompts) in a session, by the end of Session 4 with 95 per cent accuracy.

- James will display patience when waiting for John's response to an instruction. He will wait for up to one minute with one visual reminder (facilitator will tap a 'wait' symbol) in a session, by the end of Session 8 with 95 per cent accuracy.

- James will seek confirmation from his build partner by asking 'Is this right?' with 95 per cent accuracy.

The principles of SMART targets should be followed (see Chapter 8). These then helped us to choose where to start with target setting. The process is detailed below.

The targets above are all written to be: **S**pecific, **M**easured and **T**ime bound.

A for Attainable: As James already knows the concept 'next to' it was decided that 'beside' would be a good word to select. 'Next to' can be used as a synonym to 'beside' to explain its meaning. We felt this meant that James would be able to achieve this target within a couple of sessions. This rapid progress is very motivating for a child and will ensure his future engagement in the sessions.

Fading prompts will be used to gradually increase the length of time James is able to wait for a response without adult intervention. We will explain to John why James requires time to process language and respond. Our experience has shown that prompts, tokens and the motivation of building with LEGO® bricks make this an attainable target. Tokens will be rewarded very frequently for any waiting period. Initially we may give tokens every two seconds. We would then gradually increase the length between tokens to extend the waiting period.

James seeks confirmation from an adult. This suggests that seeking confirmation from a peer is attainable.

R is for Relevant: 'Beside' is a word often used within the curriculum so is a relevant target to increase access to many lessons.

James's lack of patience is a barrier to his social progress in all settings and is therefore a very relevant target.

Seeking confirmation from a peer is an important step in accepting feedback from others. It is the first step in monitoring if the communication process is working (the first step of the communication repair process).

Choosing a build partner

The build partner would need to have a better use of language (Bloom and Lahey, 1978). This will allow them to function as a role model for social use of language.

John and James were felt to be compatible build partners based on their targets, their similar cognitive abilities and chronological age.

Prompts

As most of the aims for James are based on the social use of language, all prompts will be used initially and will fade from spoken and visual, to just visual and then no prompt.

Choosing a model for John and James

It is important that the first model can be completed within one session. It also needs to be simple in design to ensure the first session is socially enjoyable and within John's attention range. Models will be gradually increased in length as James's patience and John's attention control increases.

It was decided that we would carry out the initial session using a 12-step model using DUPLO® for speed and motivation. This model was a small house with a figure and a dog. John had recently been given a puppy for his birthday and so was highly motivated by this build. James likes the repetitive pattern of windows.

All bricks in this model will include colours and shapes that had been mastered by both children.

The facilitator must provide a choice of small and large bricks so these terms can be used to meet John's targets. If the simple model does not contain the correct range of bricks you can 'cheat' by adding some extra bricks from another model (this could be a LEGO® brick).

The build will need to include directions to place bricks 'in front of' others. Therefore, the sequence of the build is important, i.e. start at the back of a build and build forwards. The build also needs to include the term 'beside' to meet James's language target.

Initial session

The Building Language Using LEGO® Bricks session is explained and rules are generated (see Chapter 7).

The targets for each child will be explained and the build partner's role in helping achieve these is outlined, for example James will say 'large' instead of 'big' to help John learn this word.

Prompts

John was given symbols for:

- large

- in front of

- all the colour symbols (these colour symbols are used to reduce a 3 ICW instruction to a 2 ICW instruction if needed).

James was given symbols for:

- beside

- wait

- is it right?

(We have not included a 'wait' symbol in the resources as these vary with each child. We have successfully used the amber symbol from a traffic light system. We have also used a clip art 'wait' picture.)

Points for the facilitator to note

The facilitator will need to manipulate the brick choices offered to John to ensure that some are at a 3 ICW level. If he struggles with this, a colour symbol can be used to reduce the pressure on his memory (see Chapter 6). If you point to the colour symbol as you say the word this negates the need for John to hold that word in his auditory memory, as he has the visual image to help. So 3 ICW 'Get the *big, blue square*' becomes 2 ICW 'Get the *big*, blue (plus visual image) *square.*'

The facilitator will need to offer choices of large and small bricks and ensure that James uses the word large instead of big. In some models there may not be a choice of big and small bricks of the right colour. The facilitator can 'cheat' by mixing in some bricks from another model to ensure the right options are on the table.

The facilitator will remind John to use the word 'beside' instead of 'next to' (by using a symbol with the word 'beside' written underneath and by verbally modelling this for him). It is useful to discuss with the children how they can support each other at the beginning of the session.

The children will initially be sat next to one another to help understanding of 'in front of' from the same perspective. They can be moved to opposite sides of the table to build a greater understanding of this concept once the initial target is achieved.

James will be prompted to wait for John's response by tapping the 'wait' symbol and saying, 'wait'. Waiting will be immediately reinforced with a token. Several tokens can be given for one waiting period to establish a longer wait. The time of the wait will be gradually expanded. Prompting will then reduce to just tapping the symbol. The number of tokens during a wait will gradually reduce.

James will be prompted to ask for confirmation by the facilitator tapping the 'is it right?' symbol and saying, 'Ask John if it's right.' In our experience the children often ask the facilitator if they are right. This then needs to be redirected to John: 'Ask John.' The facilitator can also use signing or pointing to prompt this.

Progressing skills

As targets are achieved, new targets can take their place or the target can be taken to a higher level, for example, including a different perspective by moving the children to opposite sides of the table.

Models should gradually increase in length and complexity as skills build.

The facilitator should intervene less and less as skills build.

Using Building Language using LEGO® Bricks with non-verbal or pre-verbal children

Some children are classed as non-verbal if they do not have the oral skills to produce speech sounds. These children may understand language and be able to formulate sentences in other forms but cannot produce speech. Others may produce attempts at speech sounds but their speech is so unclear that all but those very familiar to them cannot understand their attempts. These children require what is called Alternative and Augmentative Communication strategies (AAC).

Some children on the autism spectrum understand language and have a wide vocabulary stored in their memory but do not use verbal language to communicate (Blackburn, 2012). They rely more on gesture, routine and non-verbal communication and sounds.

Building Language Using LEGO® Bricks can be used to facilitate the use of AAC strategies for children who require this to augment their speech attempts or to replace speech where this is needed. For pre verbal children on the autism spectrum these AAC strategies can form a step towards the use of verbal language.

AAC strategies can include:

- the use of manual signing (see Chapter 6 for details)

- the use of visual images including, symbols, photographs or drawings (see Chapter 6)

- the use of Voice Output Communication Aids (VOCA). These are electronic devices that can produce a spoken word or phrase.

Our experience has been to use a selection of all of these approaches with children who require AAC strategies.

This intervention is a powerful and motivating way of developing the skills needed to be a successful AAC user. For example:

- learning to locate relevant symbols or learning to produce the correct signs

- learning to judge which system is most appropriate for their listener and the situation

- learning how to gain and keep a communication partner's attention whilst you construct an instruction

- learning to repair communication breakdown

- learning how to question or clarify an instruction
- learning social niceties like greetings, goodbyes etc.

We have included visual aids that can be used as AAC strategies or prompts in the appendices of this book.

Conclusion

Building Language Using LEGO® Bricks is an intervention that takes its origins from the inspirational work of Dr LeGoff and Gina Gómez de la Cuesta *et al*. Our evidence base for its effectiveness is purely clinical. We would welcome formal research to provide objective evidence for what we have witnessed in our sessions.

Building Language Using LEGO® Bricks is a fun and motivating way to develop fundamental skills that are the building blocks to communication.

It can be used to target the development of understanding and use of basic concepts, understanding and use of longer and more complex sentences and the social communication skills needed to become a competent communicator.

Sessions provide intensive exposures to targeted skills within a short space of time, in a naturalistic setting.

Our aim is that this book gives you an in-depth understanding of how to use this intervention with the children in your care.

We have adapted sessions according to children's needs, motivators and skill levels. We hope that we have given you the basic tools to use it flexibly and adapt it for your needs.

The evolution of Building Language Using LEGO® Bricks has been a gradual process. It has been both exciting and thought provoking for us. Our initial sessions were very different from the current approach. The children, their families and the staff we have trained have taught us a great deal about how to maximize the results of this intervention in as short a time as possible.

We hope that you enjoy the sessions as much as we have and that you continue to develop it to suit the needs of your child.

APPENDIX 1: ASSESSMENT CHECKLIST

Concept development

Colour	Pre intervention		Post intervention	
	comp	expr	comp	expr
Red				
Green				
Blue				
Yellow				
Black				
White				
Orange				
Brown				
Pink				
Purple				
Grey				
Light				
Dark				

Shape	Pre intervention		Post intervention	
	comp	expr	comp	expr
Square				
Rectangle				
Triangle				
Circle				
Slope				
Curve				
Semi circle				

Size	Pre intervention		Post intervention	
	comp	expr	comp	expr
Big				
Little				
Large				
Small				
Long				
Short (length)				
Thin				
Fat				
Flat				
Tall				
Short (height)				
Tiny				
Medium				

Sequences	Pre intervention		Post intervention	
	comp	expr	comp	expr
Before				
After				
Start				
Finish				
Change				
First				
Next				
Last				

Position	Pre intervention		Post intervention	
	comp	expr	comp	expr
On				
Under				
Between				
In				
Next to				
Beside				
In front of				
Behind				
End				
Middle				
Corner				
Edge				
Left				
Right				
Centre				
Opposite				
Other side				
Front				
Back				
Move				
Turn				

Other

	Pre intervention		Post intervention	
	comp	expr	comp	expr
Numbers 1–5				
Numbers 5–10				
Numbers 10–20				
Numbers 20 plus				
Smooth				
Bumpy/rough				
Shiny				
Transparent/clear				
More				
Less				
Same				
Different				
Another				

Information-carrying words

	Pre intervention		Post intervention	
	comp	expr	comp	expr
1 ICW				
2 ICW				
3 ICW				
4 ICW				
5 ICW				

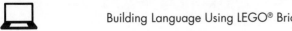

Question words

	Pre intervention		Post intervention	
	comp	expr	comp	expr
What?				
Where?				
Which?				
How?				
How many?				

Repair strategies

	Pre intervention		Post intervention	
	comp	expr	comp	expr
Gain/regain attention				
Request repetition				
Ask question				
Seek confirmation				
Ask for help from adult				
Ask for help from peer				

Non-verbal communication skills

	Pre intervention		Post intervention	
	comp	expr	comp	expr
Appropriate eye contact				
Joint attention				
Patience				
Turn taking				
Problem solving				

APPENDIX 2: MODEL CHECKLIST

Model:				
No. of steps:				
Concepts				
Colour	Shape	Size	Position	Other

APPENDIX 3A: SYMBOLS FOR COLOUR

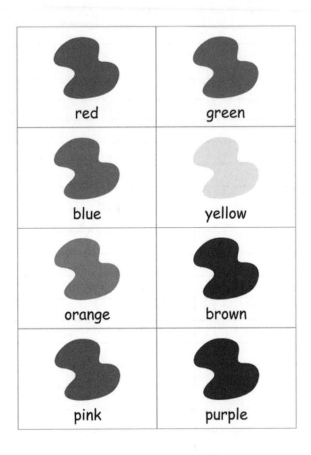

red | green

blue | yellow

orange | brown

pink | purple

APPENDIX 3B: SYMBOLS FOR COLOUR (CONTINUED)

grey	black
white	

APPENDIX 4: SYMBOLS FOR SHAPE

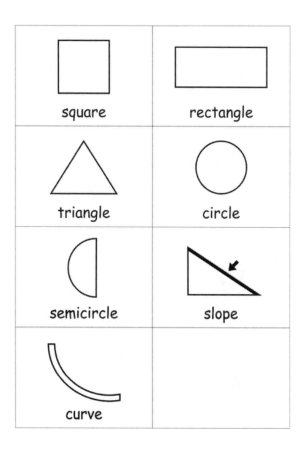

APPENDIX 5A: SYMBOLS FOR SIZE

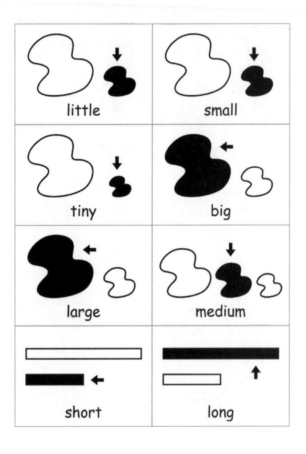

APPENDIX 5B: SYMBOLS FOR SIZE (CONTINUED)

tall	short
fat	thin

APPENDIX 6A: SYMBOLS FOR POSITION

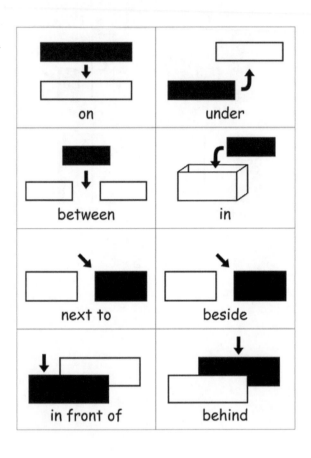

APPENDIX 6B: SYMBOLS FOR POSITION (CONTINUED)

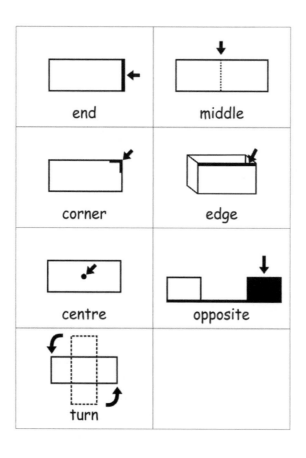

APPENDIX 7: SEQUENCE OF CONCEPTS (FORM)

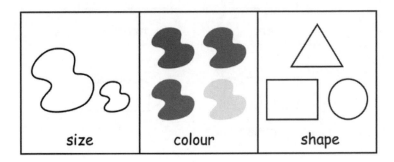

APPENDIX 8: SYMBOLS FOR QUESTIONS

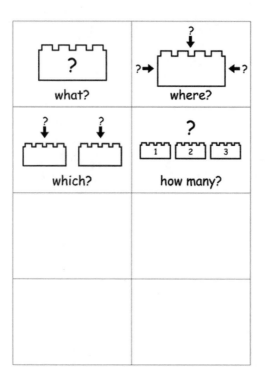

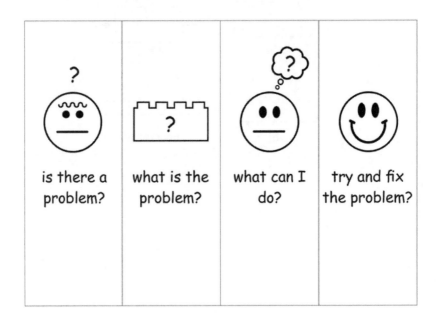

APPENDIX 10: BADGES

builder	engineer
supplier	

APPENDIX 11: TOKENS

token	token	token	token
token	token	token	token
token	token	token	token
token	token	token	token
token	token	token	token
token	token	token	token
token	token	token	token
token	token	token	token

APPENDIX 12: SESSION EVALUATION SHEET

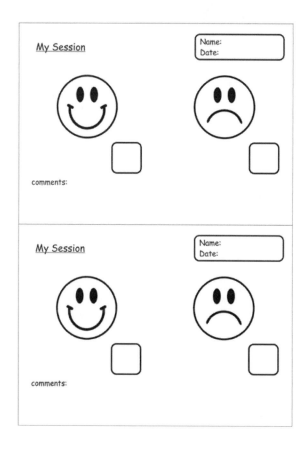

References

American Psychiatric Association (1994) *Diagnostic and Statistical Manual of Mental Disorders*. 4th edition (DSM-IV). Washington. DC: American Psychiatric Association.

American Psychiatric Association (2013) *Diagnostic and Statistical Manual of Mental Disorders*. 5th edition (DSM-5). Washington. DC: American Psychiatric Association.

Attwood, T. (1998) *Asperger's Syndrome*. London: Jessica Kingsley Publishers.

Baron-Cohen, S., Leslie, A. and Frith, U. (1985) 'Does the autistic child have a theory of mind?' *Cognition 21*, 1, 37–46.

Bates, E., Marchman, V., Thal, D., Fenson, L., *et al.* (1994) 'Developmental and stylistic variation in the composition of early vocabulary.' *Journal of Child Language 21*, 1, 85–123.

BBC Health (2013) *Baby Development 1–3 Months*. London: BBC. Available at www.bbc.co.uk/health/physical_health/child_development/babies_dev1-3.shtml accessed on 17 March 2013.

Bercow, J. (2008) *The Bercow Report: A Review of Services for Children and Young People with Speech, Language and Communication Needs*. Nottingham: DCSF Publications.

Blackburn, R. (2012) 'Logically Illogical: Information and Insight into Autism.' Birmingham University, Module: 11 11475/11 05542. 15 September 2012.

Bloom, L. and M. Lahey (1978) *Language Development and Language Disorders*. New York: John Wiley.

Boucher, J. (2009) *The Autism Spectrum. Characteristics, Causes and Practical Issues*. London: Sage Publications Ltd.

Breen, M. J. (1984) *Cognitive Patterns of Learning Disabled Students as Measured by the Woodstock-Johnson Psychoeducaional Battery.* Denver: University of Denver.

Clark, E. (1995) *The Lexicon in Acquisition.* Cambridge: Cambridge University Press.

Cooper, J., Moodley, M. and Reynell, J. (1978) *Helping Language Development: A Developmental Programme for Children with Early Language Handicaps.* London: Edward Arnold Publishers.

Ebbels, S. H. (2007) 'Teaching grammar to school-aged children with Specific Language Impairment using Shape Coding.' *Child Language Teaching and Therapy 23,* 67–93.

Enderby, P., Pickstone, C., John, A., Fryer, K., Cantrell, A. and Papaioannou, D. (2009) *Resource Manual for Commissioning and Planning Services for SLCN.* London: Royal College of Speech and Language Therapists (RCSLT).

Frith, U. (2003) *Autism Explaining the Enigma.* Malden: Blackwell Publishing.

Frith, U. (2012) 'When psychologists become builders.' *The Psychologist 25,* 8, 600–603.

Gammeltoft, L. and Nordenhof, M. (2007) *Autism, Play and Social Interaction,* London: Jessica Kingsley Publishers.

Gardner, H. (1991) *The Unschooled Mind: How Children Think and How School Should Teach.* New York: Basic Books.

Golinkoff, R. M., Jacquet, R. C., Hirsh-Pasek, K. and Nandakumar, R. (1996) 'Lexical principles may underlie the learning of verbs.' *Child Development 67,* 6, 3101–3119.

Johnson, M. and Elias, A. (2010) *East Kent Outcome System for Speech and Language Therapists.* Whitstable: East Kent Coastal Primary Care Trust.

Jordan, R. and Powell, S. (1995) *Understanding and Teaching Children with Autism.* Chichester: John Wiley and Sons Ltd.

Knowles, W. and Masidlover, M. (1982) *The Derbyshire Language Scheme.* Matlock: Derbyshire County Council.

Koegel, L., Singh, A. and Koegel, R. (2010) 'Improving motivation for academics in children with autism.' *Journal of Autism Developmental Disorders 40*, 9, 1057–1066.

LeGoff, D. B. (2004) 'Use of LEGO® as a therapeutic medium for improving social competence.' *Journal of Autism and Developmental Disorders 34*, 5, 557–571.

LeGoff, D. B., Gómez de la Cuesta, G., Krauss, G. W. and Baron-Cohen, S. (2014) *LEGO®-Based Therapy.* Jessica Kingsley Publishers.

Lillard, A., Lerner, M., Hopkins, E., Dore, A., Smith, E. D. and Palmquist, C. M. (2013) 'The impact of pretend play on children's development: A review of the evidence.' *Psychological Bulletin 139*, 1, 1–34.

Maguire, R. (2014) *I Dream in Autism.* Buckinghamshire: A Penn PR.

Matson, J., Matson, M. and Rivet, T. (2007) 'Social-skills treatments for children with autism spectrum disorders: An overview.' *Sage Publications 31*, 5, 682–707.

National Autistic Society (2009) *LEGO® Helps Social Development of Children with Autism.* London: National Autistic Society. Available at www.nas.org.uk, accessed on 18 November 2009.

National Autistic Society (2016a) *What is Autism?* London: National Autistic Society. Available at www.autism.org.uk/about/what-is.aspx, accessed on 20 March 2016.

National Autistic Society (2016b) *Changes to Autism and Asperger Syndrome Diagnostic Criteria.* Available at www.autism.org.uk/about/diagnosis/criteria-changes.aspx, accessed on 20 March 2016.

Norbury, C. F. (2016) 'Social (Pragmatic) Communication Disorder.' *Bulletin: The Official Magazine of the Royal College of Speech and Language Therapists, 22–23.*

Owens, G., Granader, Y., Humphrey, A. and Baron-Cohen, S. (2008) 'LEGO® Therapy and the Social Use of Language Programme: An evaluation of two social skills interventions for children with high functioning autism and Asperger syndrome.' *Journal of Autism and Developmental Disorders 38*, 10, 1944–1957.

Oxford Dictionaries available at www.oxforddicitionaries.com.

Stahl, S. and Nagy, W. (2005) *Teaching Word Meanings.* New Jersey: Lawrence Erlbaum Associates.

Tomasello, M. and Farrar, M. J. (1986) 'Joint attention and early language.' *Child Development 57*, 6, 1454–1463.

Vermeulen, P. (2001) *Autistic Thinking: This is the Title.* London: Jessica Kingsley Publishers.

Vygotsky, L. S. (1978) *Mind in Society: Development of Higher Psychological Processes.* Cambridge, MA: Harvard University Press.

Wing, L. and Gould, J. (1979) 'Severe impairments of social interaction and associated abnormalities in children: Epidemiology and classification.' *Journal of Autism and Developmental Disorders 9*, 1, 11–29.

World Health Organization (1993) *International Classification of Diseases.* 10th edition. Geneva: World Health Organization.

Subject Index

Sub-headings in *italics* indicate tables.

Author Index